W9-CMR-727

THE GENETIC CONNECTION

HOW TO PROTECT YOUR FAMILY AGAINST HEREDITARY DISEASE

THE GENETIC CONNECTION

HOW TO PROTECT YOUR FAMILY AGAINST HEREDITARY DISEASE

David Hendin and Joan Marks

WILLIAM MORROW AND COMPANY, INC.
NEW YORK   1978

Printed in the United States of America.

1   2   3   4   5   6   7   8   9   10

Library of Congress Cataloging in Publication Data

Hendin, David.
    The genetic connection.

    Bibliography: p.
    Includes index.
    1. Genetic counseling. 2. Genetic counseling—
United States—Directories. I. Marks, Joan H., joint author.
II. Title.
RB155.H46   613.9   77-10820
ISBN 0-688-03265-6

BOOK DESIGN   CARL WEISS

FOR
SARAH AND BENJAMIN HENDIN
AND
ANDREW, ELIZABETH, AND
MATTHEW MARKS

ACKNOWLEDGMENTS

THE AUTHORS WOULD LIKE TO THANK THE FOLLOWING individuals for their assistance in this project: Eva Beller, Arthur Bloom, Janet Bookman, Nancy and Joseph Camarano, Rose and Nick Colavitos, Gerald Dworkin, Claudia Glassman, Marjorie Guthrie, Audrey Heimler, Aaron Hendin, Sandra Hendin, Phyllis Klass, Andrew Marks, Paul A. Marks, Elinor Miller, Roberta Silman, Nancy S. Wexler, J. Benjamin Yablok, Mildred Zimelis.

Dr. Lawrence Shapiro also reviewed the entire manuscript and made valuable suggestions. Deborah Geltman's editorial criticism was important and greatly appreciated.

The contributions of all the above individuals differed greatly, but each contributed in an important way to the book and their efforts are much appreciated. The responsibility for any opinions or inaccuracies herein, however, must rest solely with the authors. In every case history, fictional names have been substituted for actual names.

CONTENTS

CHAPTER

1

WHAT
IS THE
GENETIC
CONNECTION?

IF YOU PLAN TO HAVE CHILDREN, THEN YOU MUST UNDERstand the genetic connection. The health and happiness of your family may very well depend on it.

Medical genetics is the fastest-growing and perhaps the most commonly misunderstood area of medicine today; it also may be the field of medicine most critical to your family. You can clearly grasp the importance of understanding the genetic connection when you listen to the parents of a newborn child who has come into the world with an inherited birth defect ask: "But why us?"

The answer to their question lies in understanding the genetic connection.

The vast majority of babies are born healthy. But the mathematical chances of any family's being victimized by a genetic disease are large enough so that any adult contemplating having children ought to know the basic facts of genetic disease.

THE GENETIC CONNECTION

We can reassure you by noting that, on the average, each genetic disease occurs only once in every 10,000 live births. In total, however, the incidence of genetic disease is quite high.

Some 20 million Americans today carry true genetic diseases. And about 3 to 5 percent of all live births are affected by one or more birth defects—some mild, some devastating.

Those of you who aren't used to reading about the statistics of disease might not think that 5 percent—or 5 in every 100—sounds like much of a problem. Consider, however, that even in 1952, the last big epidemic year for polio, there were 57,879 cases of that dread disease in the United States. That comes to 367.4 cases of polio per million Americans. Describe genetic disease in the same terms and 5 cases per 100 live births becomes 50,000 cases per million live births. The epidemic of genetic disease in the United States, then, is at least 100 times more widespread than was the polio epidemic at its worst! No wonder the National Foundation—March of Dimes, which largely supported work on the polio vaccine, turned its attention to birth defects and genetic diseases once polio was brought under control.

Scientists doubt that they will ever find a vaccine to halt genetic diseases. But this major public health problem could be significantly curtailed, even with the scientific and medical information already available, if only we could acquaint more people with the problems.

Thus, the earlier-mentioned statistic about the average genetic disease occurring only once in every 10,000 live births becomes more meaningful when we see the breadth of the entire genetic disease problem. Even more to the point, we must be careful to note how particular genetic diseases such as Tay Sachs disease, sickle-cell anemia, cystic fibrosis, and thalassemia have a much greater impact on individual ethnic or racial populations. Sickle-cell disease, for example, occurs in at least one of every 625 black children.

Here are some more of the statistics of genetic disease in the United States today, according to the United States Public Health Service:

—As many as half of all miscarriages are caused by gross genetic defects. This amounts to more than 100,000 miscarriages a year in the United States alone.

—At least 40 percent of all infant mortality results from genetic factors.

—Of the 3 percent of the United States population who are mentally retarded, about four-fifths are believed to carry a genetic component.

—About a third of all patients admitted to hospital pediatric wards are there for genetic reasons.

—Each human being carries between five and eight recessive genes for serious genetic defects and, therefore, faces the possibility of passing on a serious or lethal condition to each child.

And these statistics don't even take into account the many conditions that have recently been shown to have a genetic relationship, or others which are strongly suspected of having one. These include heart disease, certain forms of arthritis, diabetes, and cancer, as well as the most common mental illnesses, schizophrenia and depressive illness.

If these problems and potential problems are so

widespread, why is it that so few of us have been aware of them? Why have we not better understood their costs?—not only the medical costs but the moral and social costs as well. It takes, for example, huge amounts of money to care for an institutionalized child with a genetic disease. But who can estimate the "cost" of the anguish of a single genetically-caused miscarriage, or the unnecessary and unwanted birth of a single child with Down syndrome or Tay Sachs disease?

Although history and scientific development have no doubt been prime reasons for the relatively small amount of attention we have given to hereditary problems for so long, another, more significant reason may well be our collective—and gigantic—human ego.

"People subconsciously rebel against the notion that genetic disease is so very widespread," says Dr. Ian Shine, director of the Thomas Hunt Morgan Institute of Genetics in Lexington, Kentucky. "Darwin notwithstanding, the human being considers himself God's most perfect creation; even the evolutionist considers himself evolution's finest product, and it goes against the grain to admit the huge number of flaws one's loins can produce."

Even though he is a professional in this burgeoning field of health care, Dr. Shine has admitted to having had such a reaction himself. He recalls when he was working with the British Medical Research Council's genetic research group in 1967 when ". . . a Canadian physician, working with aborted fetuses, demonstrated that 22 percent of all spontaneous abortions [miscarriages] were associated with chromosomal anomalies. I thought, the group thought, that the man was a crackpot!"

The big question for each of us, then, is how can we know whether we, or our children, may be subject to one of these serious inherited diseases.

Not so many years ago, the answer was very simple: statistics. It was just a matter of chance how you and your offspring fared in the great genetic crap game; just like a roll of the dice, or the spin of the Great Wheel of Fortune, it could all be reduced to a simple matter of probability. That hasn't changed, of course. But today we are learning to shoot loaded dice at those odds!

With an armamentarium of newly gained knowledge and recently devised tests, physicians now can, in many cases, do more than guess about the probabilities of a genetic disease affecting a child. *All* of the known chromosomal abnormalities can be detected *before the birth* of a child. More than 60 metabolic genetic disorders can be detected *before the birth* of a child. Tests to detect carriers have been devised for some 60 diseases, and thus we can identify the healthy individual who may be carrying a defective gene that could produce a disabling or lethal disease in future offspring. It is, however, only necessary to undergo such tests when there is specific reason to suspect genetic disease.

Furthermore, medical scientists have systematically devised a series of criteria by which an individual or a couple can determine whether they are liable to develop a genetic problem of some sort. These people are said to be *at risk.*

THE GENETIC CONNECTION

If you are one of those who may be *at risk,* today there is additional help for you. Through prenatal tests, laboratory studies, physical examinations, and a review of family history, experts called genetic counselors can help prevent many types of genetic illnesses. These counselors are often physicians with a special expertise in genetics. Sometimes, too, they are specially trained men or women who are not physicians, but who work closely with them.

A genetic counselor can tell you whether you ought to have blood tests to determine the presence of specific genetic diseases. If you are expecting a child and are worried about a genetic problem, the counselor can confirm your situation—and counsel you on ways to cope with it—or allay your fears altogether.

If you are thinking of having a child, a genetic counselor can tell you the likelihood of your passing along any genetic disease to your offspring. The availability of all these services is still not as widespread as it should —or soon will—be; besides, not enough parents and parents-to-be have begun to take advantage of these important medical tools, even where they are available. It's estimated that some 15 million Americans might benefit by a visit to a genetic counselor. If you fall into any of the following categories, you are one of them:

—You are the parents of a child with a genetic disease or birth defect and are thinking about having another child.

—Your family (or ethnic group) has any history of genetic disease and you are considering having children.

—You have taken drugs, had X rays, or been exposed

to a virus (such as rubella) at or near the time of conception of a child you are now carrying.

—You are a mother-to-be older than thirty-five years of age.

—You are a pregnant woman whose mate is fifty-five years of age or older.

—You are not thinking of having children, but you may have a genetic disease yourself.

Genetic counselors will not perform miracles. They will not be able to erase the specter of genetic disease from the face of the earth, or even from your own little family. On the other hand, the genetic counselor can help you learn about any genetic problems for which you might be at risk. That knowledge is the all-important tool that will help you and your health care team "load up the dice" against a genetic "accident" occurring in your family. You move, with the team's help, from the position of a gambler to that of a fixer!

These are some of the more compelling reasons for you to broaden your knowledge in the field of human genetics. Unfortunately, in the past, a good number of rather intelligent persons have learned to "tune out" when they heard the word "genetics." It is frequently a word that evokes an avalanche of esoteric information about double helices, deoxyribonucleic acid, reverse RNA transcriptase, or a thousand other terms from the vocabulary of the molecular biologist's laboratory.

We certainly have no intention of downgrading either the importance such information may have on present or future scientific work, or its role in educating the physician or scientist in the years to come. But in reality these words play a very small part in what most of us need to know about genetics in order to understand how it affects each of our daily lives. It's unfortunate that many of the scientists who have uncovered the mysteries of inheritance have been so disinterested, and even reluctant to explain the generalities of this exciting new medical field to the people who are so dramatically affected.

And we should emphasize that one need not be faced with the prospect of a disabling genetic illness to be one of those who might be affected. Human genetics is neither mysterious nor isolated in its effects. It involves, for example, a question as universal as determining whether your soon-to-be-born child is going to be a boy or a girl. The word "genetics" is an impressive tongue twister, which simply means "He [or she] looks just like his mother [or father]." Or, tragically, "My God. What's wrong with the baby?"

Genetics plays a major role in determining what kind of person the child will become. Will it grow tall or short? Will there be a tendency to develop such illnesses as heart disease, diabetes, mental disorders, or even cancer later in life? Is there still another kind of devastating time bomb ticking inside each of the millions of cells in that child's body? Or does each cell contain a neatly packaged set of "blueprints" that destine the youngster to an unusually long and productive life, barring physical accident or unexpected disease?

Now *that's* what we want to know about genetics. Indeed, that *is* human genetics, the science of human heredity, the study of those traits and characteristics—good and bad—that are biologically passed from generation to generation, in the past, the present, and the future.

Most young men or women who already suffer genetic diseases, or who are at risk for developing genetic diseases, or who have borne or may bear children with genetic diseases, may not be interested in learning about the complex sequence of molecules called nucleic acids, in the DNA double helix—which, indeed, may be at the root of their particular problems. What people in this situation desperately do want and deserve, however, is information of a different nature. How can they cope with their disease? Can they avoid bearing children with the disease? Is there a treatment? What can health professionals do to help those with a genetic disease get along better in life or with themselves?

These are some of the questions we have set out to answer in this book. It is especially necessary because the health care professionals have sorely lagged in their ability and desire to provide this kind of information to consumers.

GENETICS: AN ANCIENT SCIENCE

Even though the rapid expansion of our knowledge about human genetic diseases has been fairly recent, man has at least had an inkling of the problems since his very beginnings. The general principles of inheritance have been observed for millennia, and broad generalizations about them have been applied to help improve cultivated crops as well as domestic animals.

Primitive writings baked into a small clay tablet in ancient Babylonia more than 6,000 years ago discuss the pedigrees of horses and indicate possible inherited characteristics. Other ancient symbols tell about the cross-pollination of date-palm trees.

In the fifth century before the common era, Greek philosopher and mathematician Pythagoras speculated that life began with the mingling of male and female fluids, originating in various parts of the body.

Later, Aristotle speculated that those fluids, referred to as semens, were actually made of purified blood. Thus, he believed that the blood itself was the chief element of heredity.

Although modern scientific knowledge has disproven his thesis rather decisively, it is interesting to note that even some of the best-educated among us still seem to have adopted Aristotle's age-old prejudices toward the blood. Why else would phrases such as "bad blood," "blue blood," or "blood will tell," lace our vocabulary even today?

Hippocrates, the ancient Greek "father" of modern medicine, also made some observations about genetics. He noted a frequent tendency for children to receive the characteristics of their parents. Hippocrates observed, for example, that "bald people are descended from bald people, people with blue eyes from people with blue eyes, and squinting persons from squinting persons. . . . at least in the majority of cases."

In the Babylonian Talmud, the fifth-century written

codification of the ancient Hebrew laws and applications, a clear reference is made to hemophilia. But more fascinating than the reference to this disease in this ancient document is the fact that scholars of long ago perceived much about the hereditary nature of the disease. States the Talmud:

> If a woman lost two sons presumably from the effects of circumcision . . . her third son should not be circumcised. . . . Likewise if the sons of two sisters had died from the effects of circumcision, the sons of other sisters should not be circumcised . . .

Thus there was a vague idea, even among the ancients, of some of the subtle aspects of hereditary diseases.

During the twelfth century, the famous Jewish physician and scholar Moses Maimonides expanded further upon the earlier Talmudic law when he wrote:

> A woman who circumcises her first son, and he dies because of the circumcision which weakens his strength; and then she circumcises her second and he dies because of the circumcision, whether it is from the first husband or the second husband, this third son should not be circumcised at the regular time [eighth day after birth], rather we wait with him until he grows and gains strength because we do not circumcise children unless they have no disease.

This statement is especially interesting because Maimonides mentions that the third son "whether it is from the first husband or the second husband" must not be circumcised if two earlier sons have died from the ritual. The physician apparently recognized that only women could be carriers of this disease, a fact which today we know to be true. Men cannot carry the gene for the disease without being victims of the disease itself. And in Maimonides' time, most hemophilia victims died at a very young age.

For many centuries people believed the ancient Greek theories of Aristotle and Hippocrates. It was not until the middle of the seventeenth century that British physician William Harvey disproved the ancient Greek concepts of inheritance. Harvey—best remembered today as the man who first traced the blood's circulation through the body—was studying the embryos of deer. Observations led him to believe that they must not have begun as tiny creatures and simply grown larger within the womb. Indeed, he found that the tiny embryos had actually originated as eggs.

By the time English naturalist Charles Darwin came along, not much more was known. In 1859 Darwin proposed his theories of evolution—theories which actually contained no further explanations of the similarities, or differences, between parents and children.

"The laws governing inheritance are for the most part unknown," Darwin concluded. "No one can say why the same peculiarity in different individuals of the same species, or in different species, is sometimes inherited and sometimes not so; why the child often reverts in certain characteristics to its grandfather or grandmother or more remote ancestor."

It remained for a little-known Austrian monk to solve some of the basic questions leading to the dilemmas Darwin had outlined. Gregor Mendel worked in an unusual laboratory—the garden of his monastery was where he performed hundreds of experiments with pea plants and flowers.

Mendel bred and crossbred pea plants which had various physical characteristics. Among them were tall plants and short plants; plants with white flowers and plants with colored flowers; plants with smooth seeds and plants with wrinkled seeds.

He bred plants with the same characteristics. And he bred plants with different characteristics. Then, in the honored scientific manner, he carefully observed the characteristics of each of the plant offspring.

Mendel was rather surprised when he found, for example, that when he bred a pea plant that bore wrinkled peas with one that bore round peas, all the resultant plants bore round peas. Logically he might have predicted that this first generation would reflect the characteristics of both parents. Instead the wrinkled-pea characteristics of one of the parents seemed to have vanished!

But when the monk bred two of these first generation hybrid round-pea plants with each other he found the wrinkled-pea characteristic hadn't vanished after all. Indeed, the offspring of this cross produced plants with both round and wrinkled peas—75 percent of the plants had round peas and 25 percent bore wrinkled peas.

It was now obvious to Mendel that the wrinkled-pea trait hadn't disappeared after all. It had, so to speak, simply gone into hiding for a generation. Mendel was quick to spot what is now accepted as a basic principle

of genetic inheritance. It is a principle that you should make special note of, since the idea behind it will crop up again and again in the discussions to come.

In fact, it is worth remembering all three of the basic laws of heredity which Gregor Mendel formulated in 1866, since whether we are talking about peas, porpoises, pine trees, or people, these basic laws are as true today as when first formulated. They are summarized as follows:

1 / Each inherited characteristic, or trait, is governed by something Mendel called a "factor." Today these factors are referred to as genes.

2 / There are two complete sets of genes in a given individual. One set of genes is inherited from each parent.

3 / Under normal circumstances, half (one set) of each parent's genes are transmitted to each child. The genes for certain characteristics may only seem to disappear in the offspring, yet they remain intact within the individual and eventually re-emerge in subsequent generations. Genes present in the set not transmitted to the offspring will not reappear in later generations. In this way, both similarities and differences between generations can be explained.

Mendel did not specify whether he believed these "factors," or genes, actually existed, or whether they were simply mathematical concepts that he had developed. At any rate, it made little difference at the time, for Mendel's discovery received virtually no recognition from either medical scientists or his fellow biologists. Mendel eventually went on to become an administrator and his work lay ignored in the scientific literature until 1900, when it was at last rediscovered and refined. From that time on, progress in genetics began to build rapidly, but never has the progress been as spectacular as that made since 1956. It was only twenty years ago that scientists finally and accurately determined that the true number of chromosomes possessed by human beings was 46. (Previously scientists thought people had 48 chromosomes in each cell.) Within only a few years that discovery led to the explanation of how Down syndrome (mongolism) was associated with an extra chromosome, and with that finding a whole new area for investigation of human disease became ripe.

Throughout the 1950s and 1960s a rapid-fire series of discoveries were made in the field of genetics—mostly in a new branch of the science called molecular genetics, to distinguish it from the "classical genetics" of Gregor Mendel.

Monumental discoveries on the molecular level have clarified and refined many theories of classical genetics. This breakthrough research has been rewarded by a series of Nobel prizes for the scientists involved. Of critical importance was the explanation by James Watson and Francis Crick of the structure of DNA, the material from which genes are actually made. This basic revelation of the now famous "double helix" structure made it possible, at long last, for scientists to understand how the genetic material in cells duplicates itself so as to pass an exact copy of its biological information on to the next generation of cells. The genetic code had now been cracked. The master blueprint for life—not only human life, but all life—had been dramatically unveiled by the basic scientists working in their laboratories around the world.

The stage was now set for the most exciting part of any drama involving medical research. Indeed, some of the players even then were concentrating on efforts to determine exactly how all this newfound knowledge might help those human beings already affected, or whose children might be victimized in the future, by the genetic diseases.

Genetic medicine has emerged as a rapidly growing and powerful discipline with an increasing ability to detect, diagnose, and treat the family of genetic diseases. Though some of those diseases remain mysteries, they are being solved by a new generation of super-sleuths at an unprecedented pace.

CHAPTER

2

PARENTS'
PRIMER
OF
GENETICS

ALTHOUGH THE STUDY OF HUMAN GENETICS IS COMPLEX, the fundamentals of human inheritance can be simplified so that they are understandable to individuals who wish to be knowledgeable about all aspects of their medical and reproductive care. The basic explanation that follows is crucial for anyone who wants to understand how parents pass their traits—both healthy and unhealthy—to their children.

First let us take a quick look at what happens inside the body upon human conception.

WHEN SPERM MEETS EGG

A woman's reproductive organs, the ovaries, are located several inches on either side of the midway point between vagina and navel. When a baby girl is born, her ovaries already contain several hundred thousand immature eggs. By the time the girl reaches puberty, the number has shrunk to about 30,000. Only a few hundred of these eggs, or ova, will be capable of fertilization in her lifetime.

From puberty on, once a month, one of these tiny eggs reaches maturity and bursts free. This is the process of ovulation; it occurs in alternate ovaries, and usually halfway through the monthly menstrual cycle—about fourteen days after the start of a menstrual period and fourteen days before the next one begins. The short period of time during which ovulation occurs, only about twenty-four hours, is the so-called fertile period. It is the time when a woman is most likely to conceive, although there is great individual variation in this timing.

When the tiny egg—even in its smallness it is the largest cell in the human body—bursts free from ovary, it floats into the abdominal cavity. It continues floating toward the mouth of one of the Fallopian tubes which connect the ovaries to the womb, or uterus—a hollow, pear-shaped muscular organ. The diameter of the Fallopian tubes is no greater than that of a human hair, but more often than not the egg is wafted right into one of them. If the egg is going to be fertilized, this is where it will most likely occur.

The egg is fertilized by sperm cells from the male. During intercourse the male partner ejaculates millions of sperm cells—the tiniest cells in the human body—into the woman. The sperm cells move through the woman's body toward the egg. Some sperm will reach the egg within only thirty minutes; others will take much longer. Most sperm never make it to the egg, but those that do surround the egg and, if fertilization is to be successful, one of them penetrates it.

As soon as the meeting between a single sperm and egg—the largest and the smallest of human cells—occurs, they fuse together to form a single cell.

Within about half an hour after the sperm and egg are thus united, the newly-formed cell divides and forms two cells. About ten hours later, these two cells divide and make four cells; the four make eight, then sixteen, and so on.

While all this cell division is taking place, the rapidly growing cluster of cells rolls along the inside of the Fallopian tube toward the womb. The journey takes about five days.

About seven days after fertilization, the tiny fluid-filled sphere of cells, now called a blastocyst, embeds itself into the wall of the womb, where it will be nourished and will grow for nine months. Already much of its destiny has been set. To be sure, the surroundings and circumstances in which the child develops and grows up will play a large part in what kind of person he or she becomes. However, a great deal of this new person's potential—physical and emotional and intellectual—already has been determined.

CHROMOSOMES AND GENES

As mentioned previously, the nucleus of every healthy human cell contains 46 threadlike strands of genetic material called chromosomes. At certain times these 46 chromosomes can be seen to exist as 23 separate pairs.

The major exceptions to this rule of 46 chromosomes are the human sex cells—the sperm and the egg. Each of these cells contains exactly half as many chromosomes as the other body cells. Thus, when the sperm, with its 23 chromosomes, and the egg, with its 23 chromosomes, unite, a new cell is created which contains all of the basic blueprints necessary to eventually develop into a complete human being. This newly-created cell contains 46 chromosomes—in 23 pairs—with half of them inherited from each parent. The new cell is a prototype for each cell that will grow in the future person's body. This is why a child can often be seen to possess certain traits of each parent. Half of a child's traits may not come from one parent and half from the other, however, because certain characteristics dominate others. We'll talk more about that shortly.

Each newly formed cell must grow and multiply billions of times within the mother's womb before a new human being is ready to be born. And in each of the myriad cell divisions, the offspring cells will contain an exact duplicate of the original set of 46 chromosomes that was formed when the father's sperm and the mother's egg first united.

There are many thousands of possible variations that can occur when the cells of a set of parents unite. Each sperm and each egg, for example, carry the potential to create a different human being. Such variations are able to occur because each chromosome is actually made up of many hundreds of genes. Genes are chemical complexes of information that govern the specific traits that a person will develop. They are each located at a particular spot on a particular chromosome. The genes are composed of a chemical called deoxyribonucleic acid, called DNA for short. The amazing thing about this complex chemical, DNA, is the way it can exactly replicate itself. And it's all submicroscopic—even smaller than the tiny solid state components which have been so publicized as being ultra, ultra-miniature!

Just as the 46 chromosomes are paired into 23 sets, so too are the genes on those chromosomes. It has been estimated that each human cell contains enough genes to govern about 50,000 separate traits. Some of these traits are controlled by many pairs of genes, but others are controlled by only a single pair of genes. By January of 1977, the *Journal of the American Medical Association* reported that scientists had "mapped," or located, about 1,200 specific genes. But advances in human genetics are so rapid that the face of the human gene map is changing quickly.

The genes account for all of our inherited characteristics—from hair and eye color, to skin shade, baldness characteristics, and components of our various internal organ systems.

Since there are so many genes within each of our cells, a few are likely to be abnormal. Indeed, we *know* that each human being inevitably carries several faulty genes. Rarely, however, do each of the two parents carry the same defective genes. Thus, when sperm and egg meet, the healthy genes from one parent frequently overshadow—or dominate—the harmful effects of the faulty genes from the other parent with which they are paired. This is why each of us can carry several potentially dangerous genes without apparent ill effects.

Incidentally, it is this fact which can often cause problems when individuals marry close blood relatives. About one-eighth of the total number of genes are identical in first cousins, for example. It doesn't take very sophisticated mathematics to show how there is, therefore, a greater chance of duplicating harmful genes when first cousins—or nearer relatives—marry. Indeed, studies have shown that marriages between first cousins produce offspring with a mental defect three times more often than would be expected among the general population. It has also been noted that there often seems to be a greater proportion of first-cousin marriages among parents of mentally retarded persons, as compared to the general population. Most matings among cousins, however, will produce normal children.

But let us return to our discussion of genes. It is significant that abnormal genes are not the only ones that can dominate or be dominated. Indeed, all of the genes are subject to this possibility, hence certain eye color, hair color, or other characteristics can be dominated by their counterparts.

In addition to the interaction of many genes, it is also probable that certain environmental factors—such as drugs, viruses, nutrition, or radiation, for example—can adversely affect the development of a new fetus.

Genetic disorders, then, can be classified into three basic groups: the chromosome disorders; the disorders caused by single pairs of genes; and the disorders caused by a number of pairs of genes and their interaction with environmental factors, called multifactorial disorders.

THE CHROMOSOME DISORDERS

Chromosome disorders are classified as "genetic" because they involve the genetic material of which the chromosomes are made. These disorders occur when entire chromosomes are abnormal, because of either their structure, their number, or their arrangement. Although they are genetic in origin, the chromosome disorders are rarely hereditary and thus they usually affect only a single pregnancy in a family. The risk is usually small that the same disease will occur in other offspring.

When a chromosome error occurs at the time of conception it can be duplicated billions of times, and will be repeated in each cell of the new being. Since there is a mistake in the blueprints, so to speak, this individual may be born with one or more defects. Significant chromosomal abnormalities are now thought to occur in about one of every 200 live births. The vast majority of these chromosome defects are harmful.

For example, scientists now estimate that as many as one-half of all spontaneous abortions are caused by chromosomal abnormalities so serious that they altogether prevent significant development of the fetus. It is, therefore, important that a couple in which the woman has had several spontaneous abortions be evaluated for such an abnormality before proceeding with additional pregnancies.

The most common of the birth defects associated with chromosomal errors is Down syndrome, often referred to as "mongolism." A common form of this disease is caused by an extra chromosome number 21. The victim of Down syndrome has 47 chromosomes instead of 46. As usual, the chromosomes occur in pairs, except the chromosomes designated as pair 21, which occur as a trio instead. Thus the medical name for this form of Down syndrome is trisomy 21.

Among the physical characteristics of the child with Down syndrome are the skin fold at the inner corners of the eyes and other facial features which tend to give the face an Oriental appearance; hence, the origin of the term mongolism to describe the disease. The person with Down syndrome also may have a large tongue and small hands with stubby fingers. Functional defects common to persons with this disorder include mental retardation, heart defects, and an increased risk of developing leukemia.

Chromosome errors such as those resulting in Down syndrome can originate with either a mother or a father of any age. However, the chances of being the victim of such errors are especially high in the offspring of women past the age of thirty-five. This may occur because a woman's eggs can get old. With each year past the age of thirty-five, the chances increase drastically that some kind of a "genetic accident" will take place during the maturation and release from the ovary of a particular egg before it is fertilized. In the case of Down syndrome, the extra chromosome is thought to originate from incomplete separation of the chromosomes when the egg is prepared for release by the ovary.

Recently there has been increasing scientific evidence that there is also some mechanism in older men that may cause an increased number of chromosomal defects in offspring of those who father children at age fifty-five or older.

Besides Down syndrome, there are many other forms of inherited mental retardation. There are as many as six million mentally retarded people in the United States. Many of their conditions are related to chromosomal defects.

Several dozen major chromosome abnormality syndromes are already known to exist, and minor chromosome errors—which cause no observable abnormalities—have been found to occur quite frequently.

Aside from the various forms of mental retardation, among the most common serious chromosome abnormalities are those that involve the sex chromosomes. These are one pair of the 23 pairs of chromosomes in each normal cell (other than the sperm and the egg which, as noted, have 23 single chromosomes). In females both of the sex chromosomes are known as X chromosomes; thus, the normal female's sex chromosomes are designated XX. Normal males each have one X and one Y sex chromosome, and thus are designated XY.

Disorders in the sex chromosomes occur about once

among every 1,100 females and once in every 380 males. The actual effects of these sex chromosome disorders on their victims can vary from the subtle to the very obvious.

In men, one of the more common sex chromosome disorders is called Klinefelter's syndrome. It occurs when a male is born with two X chromosomes and one Y chromosome (XXY) instead of single X and Y (XY) chromosomes. The disorder may be very difficult to spot in youngsters, and little is known about the development of the XXY person before adolescence. Later in life, however, the person with Klinefelter's syndrome may have abnormally small testicles, and will often be infertile. In some of these individuals there is a diminished growth of beard and body hair.

Other male sex chromosome disorders include one in which there are two Y chromosomes (XYY). These men may be abnormally tall.

One of the common sex chromosome disorders in females is called Turner's syndrome. Victims of this sex chromosome defect have only a single X chromosome (X) instead of the two X chromosomes (XX) that women usually possess.

The girl with Turner's syndrome is often short in stature and lacks the secondary sex characteristics that give girls their feminine appearance. Girls with Turner's syndrome may need special medication to help them mature sexually; even so there is a good chance that these girls will be infertile.

Another example of sex chromosome disorders is the

hermaphrodite, who possesses both ovaries and testicles, either separately or combined as a single organ.

Although sex chromosome disorders are relatively common genetic disorders, their diagnosis is sometimes difficult. Parents who suspect any abnormal sexual development in their children should consult their pediatrician or family doctor before becoming alarmed.

Many boys and men have small testicles and penises which are perfectly normal in every respect. In other words, a man's penis size, or the size and shape of sexual organs in women, is not alone sufficient cause for alarm. Speak to the doctor about your concerns privately, not in front of your child. In all probability your child is normal, and there is no sense in burdening him with your anxiety.

THE SINGLE-GENE DISORDERS

When a genetic disease is caused by faulty genes which have been contributed to the offspring by one or both of the parents, the chance always exists that the same or similar combinations of genes will occur again in subsequent conceptions by the same pair of parents. Whether or not more than one child in a family is affected by a genetic disease is determined purely by chance. The rules of chance—called probability statistics—are the only rules which can be counted upon. It is important for you to remember that these same rules of chance are in effect for each child born to you. (With the chromosome disorders such as Down syndrome, however, the risk for bearing another child with the same disorder that an earlier child suffers increases slightly.)

This chance combination can be compared to the flip of a coin. No matter how many times you flip a coin, the odds on the outcome of that next flip remain the same—a 50-percent chance of getting heads and a 50-percent chance of getting tails.

The odds may differ with particular diseases. But for all practical purposes each set of parents at risk for one of these single-gene diseases is put in the same position as the gambler who places a bet on a spin of the wheel or a roll of the dice. The main difference is that with knowledge and professional help from a genetic counselor, the parents can learn about the dimensions of any risk they might face and attempt to load the dice with the various techniques of modern medicine. We'll talk about some of those techniques shortly.

There are three general categories of single-gene defects, and each of the most commonly known genetic diseases falls into one of these three groups. They are: dominant, recessive, and sex-linked (also called X-linked).

In *dominant inheritance* the single, faulty gene that comes from one parent dominates its normal counterpart which comes from the other. Among the more than 1,200 diseases which are known to be dominant are several forms of dwarfism including achondroplasia; some forms of chronic simple glaucoma, the eye disease which, if untreated, can become a major cause of blindness; Huntington's disease, a progressive degeneration of the nervous system which usually does not begin to show itself until the victim is about thirty years old; a condition called polydactyly, in which a person has extra fingers or toes; and hypercholesterolemia, a disease in which victims suffer high levels of blood cholesterol which, in turn, leads to a predisposition toward heart disease.

In these conditions—as well as the others governed by dominant inheritance—the offspring of couples in which one parent is affected by the disease have a 50-percent chance of having the same disease. If both parents are victims of the same dominant genetic disease, there is a 75-percent risk of each of their children becoming victims of the same disease.

If the child of such a union *is free* of the dominant defect, then there is virtually no chance that the disease can be passed on to his or her children. The rare exception to this rule—and it is exceedingly rare—would be if there was a mutation, an unexpected change, in the reproductive cells of one of the parents. Though mutations are very rare, they nonetheless may strike anyone—whether or not an individual has had a history of genetic disease.

Recessive inheritance usually occurs when both parents seem to be unaffected by the disease, but are, in fact, *carriers* of the disease. This means that in each of the parents the normal gene takes precedence over its counterpart, the weaker, defective gene. Hence the defective gene is *recessive* to the normal one.

There are more than 940 known diseases that are passed along through recessive inheritance. Among these are cystic fibrosis (see chapter 8), the inborn errors of metabolism which we will discuss shortly, and the genetic diseases which strike hardest at certain ethnic groups. Typical of these genetic diseases are sickle-cell disease, a blood disorder that mainly affects blacks; thalassemia, a blood disease that chiefly affects persons of Mediterranean descent; and Tay Sachs disease, a nervous system disorder that primarily affects infants of Eastern European Jewish ancestry.

When two parents who are carriers of a recessive gene have children, each child runs a 25-percent risk of suffering that genetic disease. Each child also has a 25-percent chance of being perfectly normal. There also is a 50-percent chance that each child of such a union will be outwardly normal, but will be a carrier of the disease exactly as its parents are. These carriers will be capable of passing the same disease to their offspring.

If one parent is normal and the other parent is a carrier of a recessive disease, there is *no chance* that an offspring will inherit the disease itself. There will be a 50-percent chance that the child of one normal and one carrier parent will not be a carrier, and another 50-percent chance that the child will be a carrier of the disease, as is one of the parents.

You will probably hear more about one broad group of the recessive diseases which are referred to as *the inborn errors of metabolism*. This is a group of diseases caused by genetic defects that result in an abnormal enzyme or other protein in the victim's body. These altered or missing enzymes influence certain chemical reactions in the body to go awry, thus often resulting in serious disruptions of good health. Among these so-called inborn errors of metabolism are phenylketonuria (PKU), a condition in which mental retardation is caused by the inability of the body to metabolize certain proteins; galactosemia, in which victims cannot digest milk and milk products and often develop cataracts and severe liver disease; and maple syrup urine disease, in which the victims die in infancy, parents often being alerted to the disease by an odor of maple syrup in the child's urine. There are many other types of inborn errors of metabolism, all of them relatively rare.

Perhaps the most difficult to understand of the three kinds of inheritance for single-gene disorders are those which are described as *sex-linked,* or *X-linked.*

Before explaining this type of inheritance, we first must remember a basic fact: Normal women each have two X chromosomes (XX) while men have only one X chromosome along with the Y chromosome (XY). The Y chromosome is smaller than the X chromosome and it apparently carries mainly genes for the traits of maleness. Since each parent gives one of these sex chromosomes to each offspring, men will transmit their X chromosomes only to their daughters. Sons *always* receive only their father's Y chromosome. (This makes sense, after all, since, to become a male, the embryonic child must receive the XY combination, and the mother has no Y chromosome to offer her offspring.)

Sometimes genes for specific diseases are carried upon the X chromosomes. These are passed along with the genetic material which determines sex itself; hence they are called sex-linked. Since the diseases are carried upon the X chromosomes, they have also been called X-linked.

If a female carries the gene for one of the sex-linked diseases on one of her X chromosomes she will nevertheless *not* suffer the disease, since she also has a normal X chromosome to dominate the effect of the disease trait. (The vast majority of the sex-linked disorders are recessive.)

Men, however, are not so fortunate. If a man's X chromosome carries one of the defective genes he has no other, healthy gene on another X chromosome to dominate it. Instead he has only the Y chromosome, which is not active in this way.

This is the reason that sex-linked diseases affect men almost exclusively. Women are frequently carriers of these diseases, but they rarely are victims of them, since in order for a woman to actually inherit a sex-linked disease, either both her parents would have had to suffer the disease themselves, or the father would have been a victim and the mother a carrier.

Because of these characteristics, it is possible for a sex-linked disease to be passed down through several generations of a family without ever actually showing itself. Eventually, however, one of the female carriers of the disease may have a son who is affected.

Among the more than 170 known sex-linked diseases are color blindness, certain forms of muscular dystrophy, the Lesch-Nyhan syndrome (the retarded youngsters who are affected by this disease engage in severe self-mutilation), certain types of spinal cord degeneration (spinal ataxia), and one of the best known of all the genetic diseases, hemophilia.

If the woman of a couple is a carrier of a sex-linked disease, and the father is free of the disease, there is a 50-percent risk of each male child inheriting the disease. There is also a 50-percent chance of each male child being perfectly normal, in which case there is virtually no chance that he will transmit the disease to his children.

If the parents described in the paragraph above have a girl offspring, she has a 50-percent chance of becoming a carrier of the disease like her mother, and a 50-percent likelihood of not carrying the defective gene. There is *no chance* that a female child resulting from such a union will actually be a victim of the disease.

MULTIFACTORIAL DISORDERS

Genetic diseases that are neither due to specific chromosome damage nor faulty single gene-pairs are called the *multifactorial disorders*. This diverse group of genetic diseases results from the interaction of many genes with other genes and, perhaps, environmental factors as well. Although the actual statistics are not known, it is estimated that the multifactorial disorders occur in 1.7 to 2.6 percent of all live births.

Among the most devastating and common of the multifactorial disorders are those known as neural tube defects. They occur about once in every 500 births. This category includes defects of the central nervous system such as spina bifida and anencephaly.

Spina bifida is a condition in which the spinal column fails to develop properly and a hole remains in the lower back. This usually occurs in the lower spine and sometimes the membranes covering the spinal cord, and the spinal cord itself actually may protrude from the body in a condition known as meningomyelocele. Sometimes surgical procedures can correct these difficulties to a limited extent, but children with this problem may never gain control over bladder or bowels, and are sometimes paralyzed from the waist down.

Anencephaly exists when an infant is born without the major portions of its brain. Indeed, the skull and scalp are usually missing altogether, and the top of the head is open. Survival for longer than a few days, of course, is impossible.

When one of these two defects occurs in a family, there is a 5-percent chance that one of the defects will recur in a subsequent pregnancy by the same parents. It is now possible to detect these defects during pregnancy. This is discussed more fully in chapter 3.

Among the other birth defects which are believed to be transmitted as multifactorial disorders are:

Clubfoot, in which the affected foot is severely twisted at the ankle. Early treatment for clubfoot can be very effective. When a family has one child affected by clubfoot there is a risk of between 2 and 8 percent of recurrence.

Cleft lip and palate occur in about one of every 1,000 pregnancies in the United States. The defects result when facial structures do not fuse together and gaps are left in the lip, the palate, or both. Surgery and speech therapy can often restore victims of cleft lip and palate almost to normal. When parents have a child with cleft lip, there is about a 4-percent chance of recurrence, while cleft palate alone has about a 6.5-percent risk of recurrence.

Congenital dislocation of the hip most frequently occurs in girls and is a condition in which the upper leg bone does not fit well into the hip joint. The chances for correcting the defect are excellent if it is recognized and treated before walking begins.

Pyloric stenosis occurs about once in every 300 births, and is much more common in boys than in girls. In this defect the muscle that leads from the stomach to the small intestine is usually thick, and nothing can pass through it. The defect can be successfully corrected surgically as long as it is recognized in time. If a father had pyloric stenosis as a baby, there is a one-in-twenty chance that each of his children will have it. If a mother had the disease, there is a one in eight-risk for each of her children.

Beyond the general figures given, there is no specific way to determine the exact potential risk of bearing a child with one of the multifactorial disorders. These figures are based on actual birth records as opposed to calculated statistical odds. But, according to Dr. Richard Erbe, a geneticist at the Massachusetts General Hospital,

In general these disorders are associated with much smaller risks of transmission than in the [single gene] disorders, the risk of a particular multifactorial disorder occurring a second time in the offspring of a couple with one affected child or in the child of an affected parent both being about five percent.

Current medical opinion holds that a large number of man's most serious afflictions that seem to have some hereditary basis may be transmitted in this complex way. The possibility also exists that in many of these diseases the individual does not actually inherit the disease itself, but inherits a susceptibility to being more profoundly affected by environmental factors that can cause the disease. This may occur, for example, with certain allergies, atherosclerosis, hypertension, certain types of cancer, schizophrenia, other mental illnesses, some kinds of mental retardation, peptic ulcers, and kidney stone disease.

CHAPTER

3

EXAMINING
BABY
BEFORE
BIRTH

DONNA'S FIRST BABY DIED TWO DAYS AFTER ITS BIRTH. Her doctor told her that the child had been a victim of Down syndrome.

"Often children with Down syndrome live comfortably for many years, but some have serious heart defects and die quickly," the doctor explained quietly.

He also told twenty-six-year-old Donna that she was "at risk" for having other children with Down syndrome, or mongolism, because she was a carrier of a specific chromosome abnormality called a translocation (see page 165). Donna's is not the typical situation, since Down syndrome usually is not actually inherited, but is the result of an extra chromosome.

Donna had not previously known that she was a carrier of a translocated chromosome. It had never affected her own health or that of her family. But she—or her doctors—might have been tipped off previously, since Donna already had miscarried four times. Frequent miscarriage is very often a sign that there is a serious genetic defect present.

When Donna learned all this, the severe emotional

strain of losing this child, and then finding out that her own genetic makeup was the reason behind the problem, "Made me go to pieces," she recalled.

You always hear about these things happening to other people, they are statistics. You never think about what would happen if you were one of the statistics. Knowing that I was at risk for having another mongoloid baby . . . I just couldn't imagine ever getting pregnant again. I just couldn't bear the thought of having another defective baby. It became a real factor in our marriage. Ron, my husband, wanted so much to have a baby of our own. So did I. But a perfect baby is quite a bit different from a defective one. Our marriage was really suffering because of this continual bickering and arguing about another baby.

Months later, one of Donna's physicians told her about a nearby genetics center. She and Ron made an appointment to visit one of the counselors there, and for the first time the couple learned that Down syndrome could be detected long before birth, while the fetus was still in the womb.

"I was so surprised to hear about this," said Donna later.

It was like hearing about a miracle. And living in a big city as we do, I was surprised that I didn't hear about it somewhere before. I understand that it's a relatively new thing, but still it has been around already for ten years. We decided to have another baby.

It may seem rather surprising that this was the first time Donna and Ron had heard about prenatal diagnosis. But the widespread ignorance and apathy regarding the availability of both prenatal diagnosis and genetic counseling are really no surprise, especially to the doctors who are involved in this field of medical work. In his book, *The Heredity Factor,* geneticist Dr. William Nyhan, chairman of the pediatrics department at the University of California, warns prospective parents:

> It is important to ask. Do not wait for the doctor to suggest the idea. Physicians are less likely than patients to think about a genetic referral, particularly at the critical period when prenatal diagnosis can be accomplished safely.

Today the most common method of prenatal diagnosis is culturing cells obtained by a relatively simple medical procedure called *amniocentesis*. As we mentioned before, it is not really a very new procedure, having been used in a limited way since the 1930s, when its primary value was in detecting possible Rh blood problems late in pregnancy in women who had a different Rh blood factor than their husbands. Today the average cost for amniocentesis and related laboratory work is between $250.00 and $350.00. Health insurance often will cover these costs, and if one needs these tests and cannot afford them, the clinic involved frequently can make the necessary financial arrangements.

The amniocentesis procedure has evolved to one which allows physicians to spot safely and accurately about 100 different genetic diseases in the developing fetus, including *all* of the major chromosomal disorders, certain structural defects of the brain and spinal column, and scores of biochemical disorders in which specific chemicals are either missing, or present in excessive amounts that can impair the baby's development.

If the tests are positive for a particular disease, the

parents are so informed; if they so choose, they then can opt to have the pregnancy terminated by therapeutic abortion.

Thanks to this comparatively simple technique of diagnosing problems in the fetus before birth, thousands of couples like Donna and Ron, who would not otherwise have dared to risk another pregnancy under ordinary circumstances, have now had one or more healthy children. By following this procedure, other less fortunate parents have been spared the birth of a child with tragic genetic disease.

Milton and Dianne are a young couple from the Midwest who have a lovely three-year-old daughter, Judi.

"We never thought we would be so lucky," explained Dianne.

Six years ago we had a little baby girl. She was so gorgeous when we first saw her. We wanted children so much. But she soon developed Tay Sachs disease and died before she was three years old. After her death, Milt and I went to a geneticist who did some blood tests and found out that both of us are carriers of Tay Sachs disease. A lot of Jewish people are. He told us that there was a one-in-four chance that our children would have the disease.

At first I remember I was relieved, since we already had one sick baby and now we could have some normal ones. But I'll never forget that when I said that to him he said something like "chance has no memory" and that this one-in-four chance was going to hold true for *each* baby we had. But he also told us about this amniocentesis test and how we could find out ahead of time if the baby was going to have Tay Sachs disease.

I wondered if I could do it. Because I had to get pregnant again, then wait for a few months before I could find out whether the baby was going to be okay. But Milt and

I decided that the odds were really on our side. So we did it. We were so happy that day the doctor telephoned us to say that the baby would not have Tay Sachs disease. We just went out to dinner and had a bottle of champagne to celebrate. It was kind of funny, really. Here we were celebrating our baby, but we had almost five months before I was going to give birth! But it was wonderful.

Amniocentesis involves the removal of a small amount of the amniotic fluid from the womb. The procedure is performed during the fifteenth to the seventeenth week after the last menstrual period, and is most frequently done in the hospital on an out-patient basis. The time frame for this test is critical, since it is only at about fifteen weeks of pregnancy that it becomes possible to withdraw sufficient amniotic fluid from the womb. The test is performed by the seventeenth week to allow plenty of time to perform a safe, therapeutic abortion if a defective fetus is discovered. This timing also allows for a second test if the cells do not grow the first time.

First the physician locates the fetus and the placenta (which will later become the afterbirth, but is now the vital link between mother and fetus) . This is done with special ultrasonic equipment that bounces high-frequency sound waves off the fetus and produces a "sound-wave picture" of it.

Once the location of the fetus and placenta are revealed and the doctor determines the safest place to insert the needle, he may inject a small amount of local anesthetic into the mother's abdomen. Soon after the injection the area becomes numb, and the doctor then pierces it with a slender needle, which he carefully guides into the fluid-filled area surrounding the fetus. This is called the amniotic sac. It is filled with amniotic fluid, which serves throughout the pregnancy to bathe the fetus and help insulate it from the outside world. Since the fetus has already been floating in this fluid for nearly four months, a number of the fetal cells have been sloughed off and are contained in it. (The doctor takes special precautions to avoid obtaining any of the mother's tissue cells in the fluid by mistake.)

Donna recalls her first amniocentesis: "It was all so fast I couldn't believe it. The doctor inserted this very thin needle through my abdomen. It felt like a blood test—uncomfortable but not painful. It didn't take more than a few minutes and it was finished."

The doctor withdraws about 20 milliliters (roughly four teaspoonsful) of yellowish amniotic fluid and carefully transfers it into sterile tubes. These samples are then sent to the laboratory. There they are spun in a large centrifuge which forces the fetal cells to the tubes' bottoms, where they can easily be extracted in high concentrations. These fetal cells are incubated in containers filled with nutrient solutions and antibiotics to encourage the cells to grow and reproduce. When the original cells have reproduced sufficiently in the tissue cultures, scientists will have enough cells for testing. It takes several weeks for the cells to grow and reproduce sufficiently, and occasionally the cells don't "take" in the tissue culture. If this happens the amniocentesis needs to be repeated to obtain another sample. Once the growth has been successfully completed, special tests will determine whether there are any of the detectable biochemical defects present, such as a lack of the enzyme Hex-A, which indicates the presence of Tay Sachs disease. The amniotic fluid itself may also be tested for a chemical called alpha-fetoprotein. In recent years scientists have learned that high concentrations of this substance often are associated with at least two very severe multifactorial disorders of the development of the neural tube—spina bifida with meningomyelocele (a severe and often fatal malformation of the spinal cord and related membranes) and anencephaly (absence of the major portion of the brain).

The test to determine whether there are any chromosomal abnormalities, such as Down syndrome, is called a karyotype, and is actually a very organized look at a person's chromosomes. Once the tissue cells have been grown, a few cells are isolated and stained with a special kind of dye. The cells are then photographed through a very powerful microscope. The photograph of a particular cell is chosen, a photograph that shows the chromosomes scattered about the inside of the cell. This picture is then cut up and the chromosomes are arranged and numbered according to their sizes. The largest pair of chromosomes is labeled number one, and the smallest pair, number 22. The twenty-third pair of chromosomes are the sex chromosomes (two X chromosomes for females and one X and one Y chromosome for males) and are classified separately.

Beyond the definite diagnosis of a number of chromosomal and biochemical defects, laboratory studies of cultured fetal cells obtained through amniocentesis can give clues to the probability that a fetus may have one of the serious sex-linked (or X-linked) diseases (see pages 45–46). Most of the 170 or so sex-linked diseases cannot be diagnosed biochemically; but those that cannot may still be evaluated when the chromosomes of the cells obtained in amniocentesis are analyzed for the sex of the offspring.

The sex-linked diseases are carried by the mother, who doesn't actually suffer from them, since women are protected from the effects of the defective gene on an affected X chromosome by the dominant, healthy version of the same gene on the woman's other X chromosome. But the male who has an affected X chromosome has no such protection, because he has a Y chromosome instead of another, normal X chromosome. The Y chromosome carries no dominant, healthy gene to counteract a parallel gene on the unhealthy X chromosome. Thus it is almost always the males who develop the sex-linked diseases.

When a previous pregnancy or positive family history leads the physician to determine that a sex-linked disease may be a possibility, amniocentesis that indicates a female fetus can be reassuring to the parents. If it is determined that the fetus is a male, however, it will stand a 50-50 chance of having the disease. In such circumstances many parents would choose to abort a male fetus, preferring to take the chance of aborting a healthy fetus rather than to take an equal chance of bearing a male child who may be a victim of a lifelong disease such as hemophilia.

When Donna underwent her first amniocentesis, she and Ron anxiously awaited the doctor's laboratory report. The news was all good. The genetic counselor was able to report, "The baby does not have a chromosomal abnormality." Because the chromosome tests also indicated the baby's sex to the doctors, the counselor asked Donna and Ron if they wanted to know in advance what the sex of their new baby was going to be. They wanted to hear the news. It was a girl. Five months later a healthy baby girl was born. When Donna and Ron took her home, everything was ready—everything pink! There was no need to wonder about what color to paint the room, or what color clothes to buy, since the amniocentesis had provided Donna and Ron with a sneak preview of their own baby's sex.

If that sounds like a great idea, don't get your hopes up. Most doctors involved in genetic counseling and prenatal diagnosis feel strongly, at least at this time, that they don't want—and indeed lack the additional facilities—to get involved in helping parents "choose" their baby's sex via amniocentesis and abortion.

A 1975 world conference on Prenatal Diagnosis of Genetic Disorders of the Fetus, in Stockholm, reported that "The group in general is not sympathetic to prenatal sex determination with the objective of aborting the fetus if it is not of the desired sex. . . . Amniocentesis is never justified merely to satisfy curiosity."

Child psychologist Dr. Lee Salk, of the Cornell University Medical College, says:

> When people feel so strongly about the gender of their child as to abort the unwanted sex they really ought to re-examine their motivations for having children in the first place. It sounds too much like a shopping expedition rather than a natural, normal phenomenon. I cannot believe that someone who would be able to offer love and acceptance to a child on the basis of its gender—that that feeling would be sincere.

It is also worth stressing at this point that amniocentesis cannot determine whether a baby will be "perfectly healthy" and normally formed in every respect.

The procedure is designed at this time to detect *only* whether a particular defect is present. The amniotic sample is not subjected to all of the available tests for every genetic defect, since this would be both too costly and too time-consuming.

What amniocentesis and cell culture *can* do, however, is to reduce the risk for a particular defect to zero. Dr. Lawrence R. Shapiro, director of the division of medical genetics at the New York Medical College, explains, "People [who undergo amniocentesis] have to be willing to take the same risk as everyone else for all the other problems." It is ironic, Shapiro notes, that the individuals who undergo amniocentesis to detect a particular defect "actually end up with a lesser risk than the general population for the defect in question."

As recently as only a few years ago, many physicians had their doubts about the safety of amniocentesis. But a definitive study by the National Institute of Child Health and Human Development was released in 1975. It showed that, in the proper hands, amniocentesis "is highly accurate and safe" and "does not significantly increase the risk of fetal loss or injury." It is also safe for the mothers.

These conclusions were based upon a four-year survey of 1,040 women who had undergone amniocentesis in the second trimester of pregnancy, and the 972 infants who had been born to them. This "test group" was compared to a group of 992 mothers in very similar medical circumstances and their 957 children. In fact, many of the mothers in the control group were themselves candidates for amniocentesis to detect genetic problems, but they had declined to have the test performed.

Medical researchers at the nine obstetric centers where these women were patients compared the study group with the control group for various complications (such as loss of fetus, adverse occurrences during the remainder of pregnancy, premature birth) and the overall outcome of the pregnancies (condition of child at birth and its development during the first year of life).

The scientists found no significant differences between the amniocentesis group and the control group in any of the categories of the study. There were, for example, 36 fetal losses among the 1,040 amniocentesis mothers. But that number was statistically the same as the 32 fetal losses which occurred among the 992 control mothers, who did not receive amniocentesis. Diagnosis of the absence or presence of the fetal defect for which the test was performed was accurate 99.4 percent of the time.

Such results were "quite impressive," noted Dr. Aubrey Milunsky, medical geneticist at the Massachusetts General Hospital, where many of the amniocentesis samples were analyzed. "I certainly hope all physicians are now offering their high-risk patients the option of amniocentesis. According to the figures, no differences can be spotted between pregnancies uncomplicated by a needle and those complicated by the amniotic tap," Dr. Milunsky said.

Nevertheless, after the study results were announced, the National Foundation–March of Dimes estimated, early in 1977, that only about 10 percent of the pregnant women who could benefit from amniocentesis actually undergo it. Those women "at risk" who *should* take advantage of amniocentesis include all pregnant women older than 35 years, women who already have had a

child with a chromosomal abnormality, those who have
family histories of chromosome abnormalities or inherited metabolic disorders that amniocentesis can help
predict, and women who are known to be carriers of
serious sex-linked diseases.

In spite of the tremendous value of amniocentesis to
many thousands of couples in the United States, certain
"Right to Life" groups have taken adamant public
stands against it on the basis of their feeling that it is a
procedure that "promotes abortion."

As a matter of fact, amniocentesis and other methods
of prenatal diagnosis appear to actually reduce the number of abortions. Explains Dr. Arthur J. Salisbury, vice
president for medical services of the National Foundation–March of Dimes:

> Before prenatal diagnosis was possible, families at risk
> for genetic disorders could be counseled only on the basis
> of statistical odds, and many opted for unnecessary abor-
> tions. Now the great majority of those parents can be
> reassured by simply withdrawing a small amount of the
> fluid surrounding the fetus.

Evidence from a 1976 survey of fifty-eight medical
centers which provided diagnostic amniocentesis sup-
ports Dr. Salisbury's contention. The study showed that
nearly 97 percent of 3,561 women whose family histories
or advanced age caused concern about the outcome of
pregnancy were reassured by the test that the defect in
question was not present. These figures correlate with
other similar surveys.

Serious birth defects were diagnosed in only 3.5 percent of the pregnancies in which women were tested,
and only 2.9 percent of the women tested chose to have

an abortion. Thus, more than 3,400 families who had been worried about having children with severe birth defects were spared further anguish.

Although amniocentesis is the oldest and most widely used of all the prenatal diagnostic techniques, it is not the only effective test. The other methods currently available or under study involve various ways of obtaining different kinds of information—cellular, biochemical, and graphic—about the condition of the fetus while it is still in the womb. The three most widely known methods are ultrasound, radiography, and fetoscopy.

Ultrasound involves the use of high-frequency sound waves and their echoes to produce television-type "pictures" of internal organs, including the uterus and the developing fetus within it. Ultrasound is a relatively new diagnostic tool, having come into widespread use only in the early 1970s. It is an outgrowth of the sonar techniques used during World War II and perfected in the following years.

During an ultrasound examination, a small device that looks a lot like a microphone is placed against the woman's abdominal area. This little instrument emits high-frequency sound waves which are reflected at varying intensities as they strike different body structures. The returning echoes are used to paint a "sound picture" on a console screen. Each scan is taken through the body on a single plane, but the overall visual effect of a series of scans is as if a tree trunk were thinly sectioned and each piece were held up to examine the rings. There is almost no discomfort during the procedure and the average ultrasound examination takes about twenty minutes.

Ultrasound monitoring is used to provide estimates of the unborn baby's age (important in cases where the time of conception is not known). This is accomplished by measuring the size of the fetal skull. This technique can pinpoint the date of conception within two weeks. Ultrasound's application in preparing for amniocentesis has already been discussed.

Radiography involves X-raying the fetus to detect various major abnormalities, particularly those having to do with skeletal structure. X rays cannot reveal certain serious defects such as anencephaly, a condition in which a child is born without most of its brain. The conditions X rays can reveal in the fetus can often be detected as well or better by other methods such as ultrasound. (X rays are especially dangerous to a woman early in pregnancy, but can be used therapeutically as she approaches term.)

Fetoscopy is perhaps the most exciting new method of prenatal diagnosis. It involves actually looking at the developing fetus through a special, flexible fiberoptic rod that the doctor inserts into the womb. As this method becomes more sophisticated, it will be possible for physicians to actually look at the fetus within the womb to see if it has any gross physical defects. Through fetoscopy it is also possible that someday the physician will be able to safely take small samples of blood and even skin directly from the fetus. This would open the way to diagnosis of a number of serious inherited blood disorders. Although a few fetuses have already been tested using this device, the technique is still too experimental for most physicians to attempt at this time.

CHAPTER

4

WHAT IS
GENETIC
COUNSELING?

IF YOU ARE FORTY-ONE YEARS OLD AND TEN WEEKS PREGnant, *you need genetic counseling.*

If you have a brother who has hemophilia, but seem healthy yourself, *you need genetic counseling.*

If you have cystic fibrosis and want to have children, *you need genetic counseling.*

If you have already had a child born with a physical or mental abnormality, *you need genetic counseling.*

Ninety percent of the people in the United States who could benefit from genetic counseling do not receive it. A major reason for this is that such individuals don't know enough about the inheritance of diseases to realize they need the advice of experts in genetics.

The small percentage of Americans who need genetic counseling and get it usually do so only *after they have already given birth to one or more children suffering from a genetic disease.*

THE GENETIC CONNECTION

When people do not get the expert help they need, the result is unnecessary tragedy for those who would have chosen to direct their reproductive lives differently if they had been given a choice.

Margaret Sonoma is one of those people who made the choice. Margaret and her husband had two healthy teenage children. They thought their family was complete . . . until Margaret found herself unexpectedly pregnant at age forty-one. Her husband, Bill, was forty-six.

At first the Sonomas were upset to discover that a new child was going to intrude on their family life. But before long they had become quite pleased at the prospect of a new baby in the family.

Margaret remembered that she had read in her local newspaper about a test for older pregnant mothers to show if their gestating child was destined to be retarded. Both she and Bill agreed that this test would be a sensible one to take, so Margaret telephoned her obstetrician for an appointment.

After giving his patient a complete physical examination Dr. Porter confirmed the pregnancy.

Margaret asked: "Do you know about this prenatal test they take on pregnant women who are my age?"

Dr. Porter seemed surprised at the question, but replied that, yes, he did know about it. "It's called amniocentesis. Do you think you need to have it?" he asked.

"Well," Margaret said, "I understand it is for older mothers, and I'm forty-one, so I thought I should have it. What do you think?"

"It's probably a good idea. Let me call the Medical

Center and find out how to arrange it for you."

The next day Dr. Porter called Margaret to tell her that the test could be done when she was in about her sixteenth week of pregnancy, but that she should call the Genetic Counseling Department now for a preliminary appointment at which the procedure would be explained. Bill and Margaret both went in for the preliminaries, and when the sixteenth week arrived they went in for the amniocentesis itself.

Twenty days after the fluid had been withdrawn from Margaret's uterus, the genetic counselor called the Sonomas and asked them to come in to discuss the results. They made an appointment for the next day.

Both Dr. Norton, the physician who had performed the procedure, and Ms. Hewitt, the genetic counselor who had explained the test to the Sonomas, came to the meeting.

Dr. Norton began: "The cells we removed in the fluid grew on schedule. We have finished our studies on them. Unfortunately, we have found that there is an extra chromosome number 21. This indicates that the baby will have Down syndrome. Perhaps you know this disease as mongolism. I must explain to you that this means your child will be mentally retarded."

Mrs. Sonoma was too shocked to reply, but her husband nodded his understanding.

Gently, Dr. Norton reminded the couple that they had two alternatives to decide upon within the next few weeks. They could have a legal abortion, or they could plan for the birth of the child with Down syndrome.

"I know it's difficult for you to accept this news right

now," said Dr. Norton. "Ms. Hewitt or I will answer any questions you have, now or later, as you are trying to make up your mind what course to follow."

Dr. Norton waited a few moments to see if there were any immediate questions. As he left the room he added, "I'm sorry to have to give you this kind of news. Please let me know if I can help you further."

"Thank you, doctor," Mrs. Sonoma mumbled. As the physician left the room Margaret looked at her husband for the first time during the session, and she burst into tears.

Although close to tears himself, Bill Sonoma held his wife quietly.

Ms. Hewitt asked if they wanted to be alone, but both of them shook their heads. Bill asked if she could explain why this terrible thing had happened.

"We can't exactly say what went wrong," the genetic counselor replied. "But we know that mothers older than age thirty-five have a much greater chance of having children with an extra chromosome 21. Since your detailed family history shows no evidence that Down syndrome runs in your family, it must be an 'accident.' "

"Are you certain that the baby will be retarded?" Margaret asked.

"Yes," Ms. Hewitt replied. "We don't know the extent of the baby's retardation, but it seems likely that he or she will be dependent on someone else's care for a lifetime. The child may live to be fifty or sixty years old. Some patients with Down syndrome can be trained to be quite self-sufficient, but others cannot be trained at all. We have no way of knowing the degree of the problem in advance."

"If we decide to have an abortion," Bill asked, "where and when will it be done?"

Ms. Hewitt said she could make the necessary arrangements at that hospital, or that the Sonomas' own physician could do so. "It should be done soon. But I think you both will need some time to discuss this with each other and think about it. Please don't try to make up your mind right now."

"But I already decided I couldn't have a retarded child," Margaret said. "It wouldn't be fair to the two boys."

"I understand how you feel, Mrs. Sonoma. But it's really important for you to have some time to think about such a decision and to make certain that it is the best one for you and your family," Ms. Hewitt said.

"Yes," said Bill. "I think Ms. Hewitt is right. Margaret, we'll go home and talk it over and then we will call her back."

"Good grief, Bill," Margaret said. "What will we tell the boys? Should we tell them the truth? What do other parents say, Ms. Hewitt?"

"It's much easier to tell the truth, Mrs. Sonoma, otherwise you may find yourself making mistakes and forgetting what you have said. You know your own boys best and can probably guess how well they will be able to accept whatever you tell them," Ms. Hewitt said. She continued, "It's not easy to tell a child that you may not want to keep the child from this pregnancy because it is not perfect. On the other hand, most children understand what Down syndrome implies. You have a lot to talk about in the next few days. Please call me if I can give you any information that will help you make your decision."

The Sonomas did telephone two days later to ask about abortion procedures. They also wanted to know whether this event meant that their sons had anything to worry about when they became parents.

Ms. Hewitt was able to reassure them that their sons would have no greater risk than anyone else of producing a child with a genetic defect.

Ultimately—within a week—the Sonomas decided to abort the fetus. Mrs. Sonoma's obstetrician performed the abortion.

The episode was emotionally draining for the entire family, but even the two teenage boys shared their parents' feeling that to knowingly bring a retarded child into the world was not right for them. The older boy, a high school student, was especially interested in the social problems of Down syndrome children and discussed them with his parents.

The type of preventive genetic counseling which the Sonomas underwent is ideal. It is most unfortunate that it is not sought by more parents who could benefit.

Another couple, Arthur and Betty Crosby, were not as fortunate as the Sonomas. They were not referred for counseling until after their second child was born. The couple's first child had been born when they were in their late twenties and had been married for several years.

At birth that first child, named Karen, appeared to be perfectly normal. But before she was one year old she began to develop symptoms that were later diagnosed as those of a genetic disease called Hurler's syndrome. By the time Karen was eighteen months old she had become "strange" to look at, she could not see properly, was obviously retarded, and had trouble breathing.

The family's pediatrician explained that Karen's condition would become progressively worse and she would probably die from the complications of the disease's effect on her body. The doctor was able to arrange to have Karen placed in a hospital that specialized in caring for children with severe genetic defects.

Even though it took several years for the Crosbys to again begin to think of having another child, they were strongly encouraged to do so by both their obstetrician and their pediatrician.

Both doctors assured the parents that this condition "could not happen again" to them.

After this advice, Betty Crosby became pregnant three-and-one-half years after Karen had been born, and in 1975 she gave birth to a second daughter, Terry.

In spite of the assurances from the doctors, Betty had been a "nervous wreck" during her pregnancy. If she had been told about prenatal diagnosis, the burden on her might have been eased by indicating that her baby did or did not have the same condition as her first daughter.

However, Betty had not been told about the test. And after Terry's birth, the parents' joy at what seemed to be a healthy baby was short-lived. Terry, too, had Hurler's syndrome and soon became mentally retarded and physically deformed.

As one might imagine, genetic counseling for the

Crosbys was an emotional affair. After Terry was born, the Crosbys demanded that their doctor get them the advice of a specialist. By the time they arrived at the consultation they were upset and not too confident that the genetic counseling team would be much more reliable than their previous doctors had been.

The Crosbys were both tense with each other. Arthur imagined that he was to blame, if not for the disease itself, then certainly for allowing his wife to become pregnant a second time. Betty, on the other hand, assumed that there was something "really wrong with me that I can only have these weird babies." The couple couldn't easily talk about their inner feelings, even though they talked a lot about what had happened to them.

Before the genetic counseling session, Betty had talked to Mrs. Linder, the genetic counselor, to arrange for all the hospital records of their babies to be sent to Dr. Johnson, the geneticist.

As soon as the Crosbys sat down for the counseling session, Betty became quite nervous and uncomfortable. She wondered whether she would have to be examined by the doctor, or if any blood tests would be taken. It was all so strange.

When Dr. Johnson spoke he explained that they had obtained most of the necessary records on the two children, and it seemed clear that the diagnosis of Hurler's syndrome was correct.

"Do you know what causes this disease?" he asked the Crosbys.

Arthur replied that they thought it happened because

the children couldn't produce an enzyme that was needed for their bodies to function properly.

"That's right," Dr. Johnson said. "What we want to find out now is how this happened, so we can understand what your chances are for having healthy babies. Do you plan to have more children?"

"Not if they can't be healthy," Betty quickly replied. "I couldn't go through it again."

"I certainly understand how you feel," the doctor said. "Today, though, we need to do two things that will be important in working this out with you. First we need to take a detailed family history from both of you which will include information about your families as far back as a few generations. Please try to remember as much as you can and understand that we may be dealing with a situation here that is important to others in your family, too. Mrs. Linder will work on this family history—what we call the pedigree—with you. Secondly, I would like another blood test taken on Terry."

After the physician left the room, the genetic counselor helped Arthur and Betty draw their family tree or pedigree.

"It was really hard to remember things so far back," Betty later recalled.

But it's amazing to see your whole family pictured on a piece of paper. If it weren't so serious it might have been fun. While we did the histories we also had a chance to ask some more questions about how we could both be healthy but still have these bad genes which made our children so sick.

The counselor explained how this particular disease was "recessive" and could only show up in children if both parents contributed to it. It suddenly dawned on me that if I hadn't married Arthur this never would have happened. What a shock! I suppose he was thinking the same thing.

It was at this point that Mrs. Linder explained to the Crosbys that there was a three-to-one chance that each of their babies would be okay.

"You mean there will always be a twenty-five percent risk that our babies will have Hurler's syndrome?" Arthur said.

The genetic counselor replied, "Yes."

Although the Crosbys were upset at this news, they were, at the same time, relieved to have found medical advice that seemed so competent.

During their next visit with Dr. Johnson, Betty and Arthur learned that the diagnosis of Hurler's syndrome had been confirmed and that both of them were considered to be carriers of the gene for this condition.

Most important, however, Dr. Johnson explained to the couple that any future pregnancies could be studied by amniocentesis and cell culture at about the sixteenth week of pregnancy. This test would show whether the fetus was producing the right amount of the all-important enzyme. If it was not, the child could be aborted with the hope that the next pregnancy would not be affected.

This was the first glimmer of hope for the Crosbys, and again they began to consider the possibility of having children—healthy children. The knowledge of this possibility changed their lives.

WHAT IS GENETIC COUNSELING?

The stories of Arthur and Betty Crosby, and Bill and Margaret Sonoma, clearly illustrate some of the problems couples may face when they seek genetic counseling. Although genetic counseling is similar to other fields of medicine, it is also very different.

"CHECKING OUT" THE FAMILY

Some families admit that they have sought genetic counseling simply to "check out whether we are normal."

There is nothing at all wrong with such a motivation. However, these families usually perceive the genetic counselor as one who will give them a definite "yes" or "no" answer to questions about their genetic health, much as the traditional physician will tell them that they "should" go on this diet, or have that operation, for example. When the genetic counselor offers answers that merely outline the possibilities of what *could* happen, the clients may become confused or even angry.

Who goes to genetic counselors for these "genetic checkups"? As we noted earlier, it is usually the family that already has had a child with a suspected genetic disease, and they seek counseling about their chances with respect to any future children they might conceive.

Genetic counseling is recommended for families with a known genetic defect of any kind, or when more than one family member is affected with the same abnormality. Other indications of the need for genetic counseling are two or more previous miscarriages, or stillborn births, sterility that is not clearly due to physical factors, and the potential mother's age being greater than thirty-five or the father's being greater than fifty-five.

There are an increasing number of couples who have a vague understanding of the role inheritance may play in reproduction who now seek counseling prior to starting their families. This is, of course, the ideal time to do so. Unfortunately, present resources in clinical genetics are not adequate to serve all prospective couples who may wish to take advantage of such preventive measures. This type of broad genetic counseling could—and perhaps even should—be handled by family physicians. At this time, however, as we clearly saw in the case of the Crosbys, many such physicians have neither the proper training nor the time to undertake this sort of counseling. In the future it is hoped that they will be better prepared to offer this reproductive counseling. There are advantages to having the family physician undertake genetic counseling. Consultation with a physician who knows the patient and the patient's family makes it easier for the patients to ask personal or possibly embarrassing questions, or questions which may reveal their lack of knowledge.

Individuals who seek genetic counseling often do not realize that in most cases the genetic counselor cannot offer definitive answers. Instead, the answers almost always will be in terms of the statistical odds or probabilities that a child born to the couple will have—or will not have—a specific genetic disease.

When a family is told that with each pregnancy they may have a 25-percent risk of bearing a child with a profound genetic illness, should this be considered a high risk? Or is 50 percent the highest acceptable risk for them? Couples often expect to be told that they have either absolutely no risk at all, or that they have a very great risk for bearing a genetically defective child. Many are surprised indeed to hear from the genetic counselor that he or she will provide only information, and that the couple must decide for themselves whether the percentage of risk is high, low, or worth gambling about at all.

THE GENETIC COUNSELOR

Today's medical genetic counselor is usually a pediatrician or internist who has specialized in treating hereditary disorders. In large medical centers, where such specialists often practice, they are usually part of a team which includes individuals with expertise in the laboratory aspects of diagnosing genetic disease, others who are diagnosticians, and still others who concentrate on helping families understand what the diagnosis may mean to them. All these specialists may be called genetic counselors. Genetic counseling may be described in many different terms which can make it confusing to those who seek help. Some services are called by these titles: "Birth Defects Center," "Developmental Disabilities Clinic," or "Genetics Unit." Whatever the name, however, most genetics units are able to refer patients to the proper service within the hospital.

THE COUNSELING INTERVIEW

The first step in arriving at an assessment of an individual's genetic makeup should be to explain what the counseling will be like and what it can accomplish.

Next both a medical history and a detailed family history, called a pedigree, are taken by the geneticist or one of the associates. If an individual who is affected by a particular disease in question is involved, a physical examination may be conducted at this time. Laboratory studies are usually necessary to confirm a suspected diagnosis. Among the tests required may be a blood test or a skin test. The results of these tests are often not available for two to three weeks. Sometimes other medical specialists may be consulted by the genetic team before a firm diagnosis can be made.

Family medical records may have to be searched out and gathered, and it is important for the patient to be forewarned that if he or she must follow this route, other family members may oppose such a procedure as an "intrusion of family privacy." Sometimes such requests are interpreted as attempts to "blame" other family members for the suspected condition. Relatives may want to follow the "what we don't know can't hurt us" theory, and therefore consciously avoid any probing into these matters.

Yet such a search can be valuable not only for the individual seeking counseling, but for the entire family. Sometimes whole family conferences are called with physician-counselors in attendance. One such gathering in 1971 focused on the extended family of Kenneth Swier of Colton, South Dakota. Swier suffered from spinal cerebellar degeneration, a fatal hereditary nerve disease that attacks the central nervous system. First the disease affects balance and coordination, then it impairs speech, and finally it makes it impossible to breathe. The disease has about a fifteen-year timespan, at the end of which its victims usually die of pneumonia.

Spinal cerebellar degeneration is a dominant disease, and thus it can be passed along only by those parents who actually have it—and 50 percent of their offspring are likely to develop the disease themselves. Unfortunately this disease cannot be detected until it actually begins to appear, and thus many of its victims already have had children before they find out they are affected.

Most of Ken Swier's sixty-one relatives who lived near him at the time he became ill tried to avoid thinking about the possibility that this family curse would affect them.

But some members of Swier's family sought the help of the National Genetics Foundation [NGF], which stepped in to do some detective work. The family disease was traced back as far as Ken Swier's great-great grandfather, Gerritt John Vandenberg, a Dutchman. Some of Vandenberg's children had emigrated to the United States from Holland several generations ago.

The NGF staged a reunion for ninety-five of the Dutchman's descendants, whom they had located in five states and Argentina. At the family gathering, a number of physicians were able to trace six hundred individual descendants of great-grandfather Vandenberg. They thus compiled one of the most complete genetic records ever recorded of a single family.

In a series of examinations, the physicians found possible early signs of the fatal disease in twenty of the family members present. All those who attended the gathering were counseled with regard to their risks, and in this case the physicians advised those in line to develop the disease not to have children, or at least to delay starting their families until they were certain they had escaped the family's fatal inheritance.

While group counseling of this sort is indeed dramatic, it is especially important that individual family members have an opportunity to receive counseling help as well. This more private counseling allows individuals to deal better with their own concerns and helps insure that each person understands the disease and its reproductive implications.

Even in the case of a single couple's genetic counseling, repeated visits may be necessary in situations where the diagnosis is not clear-cut or where the couple simply needs more help in dealing with their problem.

An important example of the need for additional genetic counseling would be in the case of a sex-linked condition. Anxiety about one's own children is often so intense that a woman who gives birth to a child with hemophilia, for example, may not even hear her doctor's suggestion that her sister should also be concerned about being a carrier of the same troublesome gene. But in the weeks following the initial counseling the woman and her husband may begin to have questions about the rest of their family and may want to seek additional counseling to answer them.

Also, parents who have learned they will have a diseased child, but have chosen not to have an abortion, may seek more counseling to learn how to best handle their child once it is born and what community resources will be available to them.

WHAT IS GENETIC COUNSELING?

HOW PATIENTS REACT

The period of time it takes before the geneticist is able to give his or her assessment to the concerned individuals can be an agonizing period. Patients are often so tense that they are unable to listen carefully to what is said to them when the diagnosis is finally offered. Another common reaction is for the patient to hear the diagnosis perfectly, but to fail to grasp the significance of what has been heard, or even to fail to grasp the long-term implications for the individual or the family group. Such reactions are not at all unusual and families should be encouraged to return for additional counseling or to ask more questions whenever they are confused. Sometimes a letter from the doctor detailing the diagnosis and explaining once again how it was determined helps to clarify the situation for those who sought the counseling.

Since there are more than 2,000 known genetic diseases, ranging from the nearly insignificant to the devastating, the spectrum is so broad that it is not easy to be specific about how "most" people react to the possibility of carrying such a disease potential. Almost every potential victim of inherited disease, however, feels some degree of societal stigmatization because he or she is "different" from what is considered normal. Nearly all individuals who are told that they carry the potential of passing along a genetic disease experience some degree of anger, fear, depression, or social withdrawal when they learn about this "difference." These

are all common, normal, and hopefully temporary reactions.

Susan, a twenty-two-year-old woman who was at risk
for Huntington's disease, considered herself "defective"
because of her susceptibility. This affected the way she
perceived her relationships with men. Susan was frightened that any "ideal" man would not really be interested in her because she was not normal in a genetic
sense. Thus, in her fantasies, she chose an ugly man,
relating his outward ugliness with what she saw as her
own inward ugliness. In other words, she felt equal
with an ugly man, but with her "ideal" man—even in
her fantasies—she felt ashamed of what she thought to
be her "defect."

Another kind of reaction can be seen in Fran, a
twenty-eight-year-old woman who had just learned that
her mother had suffered from Huntington's disease.
Fran already had two small children and now for the
first time was told that she had a 50-percent chance of
developing the same disease that had caused her mother
to suffer so greatly. And if Fran did develop the disease,
she was told that each of her children also had a 50-
percent chance of becoming victims of Huntington's
disease.

"I went through a bad depression for about two
weeks," Fran recalled.

> I'd sit there and cry because I'd think of how I might miss
> everything my mother missed. She never saw us married
> or have kids. I want to be a grandma. . . . I told my hus-
> band I wanted a divorce so he could get out of the legal
> stuff—let the state take care of me. . . . What really got

to me was the kids and how much of their lives I'd miss, depending on how old I was if and when I got it. I'd cry if I thought of any of their graduations or getting married. Anything like that would bring on a tear jag. And, of course, me not being there mainly for both of them. Then, after two weeks I just snapped right out of it like I went into it. I've never given it another thought.

Some people, such as Fran, will try to fool themselves into believing that they are able to forget this kind of a burden. Most individuals, however, know they cannot "forget" and, like Fran, many have commented on the amount of pain involved in this remembering.

A mother of a baby with Down syndrome remembers feeling as if "my body had betrayed me. I was totally undermined in my sense of myself. There were just bad things in me which had to come out sooner or later. . . . It was as if the baby was a retribution for a life of sin."

THE PARENTS' GUILT

There is, traditionally, a tremendous amount of guilt involved in conceiving and bearing a child with a severe genetic defect. Not only do parents often blame themselves, they more than occasionally have severe emotional crises because of it. This can play havoc with a marriage, particularly if one parent is pinpointed as having the genetic problem, and the other parent is thought to be normal.

Each parent may experience both anger and guilt toward the other. In families which are culturally expected to have many children, the frustration of reproductive drives can be very difficult for the partners to manage.

One mother of a Down syndrome baby revealed that even after many years, she still had nightmares about the birth of her affected child. "The pain never really goes away," she said.

Sometimes this intense guilt is encouraged by an uninformed health professional—even, perhaps, by the physician. Dr. William Sly, director of the medical genetics program at Washington University, St Louis, told a 1972 symposium about a couple who had been referred to his center.

The woman appeared to be normal, but her twenty-eight-year-old husband had suffered severe damage to his nervous system at birth, due to a lack of oxygen and other physical traumas. Although the husband was normal in other respects, he was confined to a wheelchair and had obvious physical handicaps. Still, he was capable of leading nearly a normal life. In fact, at the time he was first seen by the St. Louis consultants he was in his third year of college.

"The couple's first pregnancy had produced a child that died shortly after birth with spina bifida, meningomyelocele, and hydrocephalus," reported Dr. Sly.

Their second pregnancy produced an anencephalic child that also died shortly after birth. Following the second delivery, the obstetrician charged out of the delivery suite and told the man he had no right to contemplate further children unless he had chromosomal studies to prove that he was fit.

The girl's family, strongly influenced by the physician, blamed the husband and demanded that she divorce him. The small community in which they lived began to treat the man with suspicion.

"Obviously," Dr. Sly observed, "the physician, the family and the community were ignorant of the facts and blamed this man for the neural tube defects in the offspring because of his other disability. Their cloudy judgment was nearly destroying the couple."

Ironically, in this situation, the physicians were able to show that the recurrence risk in this disorder is due equally to factors contributed by both parents. That is, the neural tube defects in the newborns were probably due to something contributed by both the mother and the father, despite his very visible disabilities and her outwardly normal appearance.

Good genetic counseling should ease the guilt that seems to accompany the birth of a defective child, by helping to eliminate the unrealistic nature of this guilt. It is not abnormal to have these feelings for a while, but once biological facts are clarified by the genetic counselor, the mother and father should then be able to discharge much of their initial fury at their bad luck through an open discussion of these normal, but very painful, reactions.

This kind of moral and emotional support is not often available even from close friends or relatives. Friends are often simply embarrassed to recognize genetic imperfections in others. They ". . . don't know what to say. They offer foolish advice hoping to be helpful." As one mother tells it: "I've tried to talk to my family about what happened to the baby. But they say, 'Don't talk about it, you'll just make yourself more unhappy. Don't even think about it,' they say. As if that were possible!"

This grief and guilt associated with either bearing a genetically defective child, or having a genetic fault in one's own makeup, must be resolved realistically. And this is one of the chief goals of the counseling process. Studies have clearly shown that even brief counseling can help a parent's damaged feelings about himself or herself.

"I CAN'T BELIEVE IT"

Susan and Harry Collins' baby was born with Down syndrome. Susan was still feeling numb late in the afternoon on the day of the birth when Laura Thompson, the genetic counselor, visited Susan to talk about the new baby.

"I know how upset you must be, Mrs. Collins. It is my job to meet with all the mothers in this hospital who have problem births."

"I can't believe it has happened to me," Susan sobbed. "Yesterday my only concern was to get this baby born. Not even twenty-four hours later it's like the earth caved in. I'm numb. But why me? I feel like such a failure."

"How is your husband taking it?" the counselor asked.

"He's mostly worried about me. But I don't see how I can take care of the baby. I don't even want to see it."

When Harry Collins walked into the room a few

moments later he immediately showed his concern for his wife's feelings. "How could you think it was your fault?" he asked.

Yet something in the tone of Harry's voice led Mrs. Thompson to ask if they understood how Down syndrome developed. When she explained how each parent contributes the genetic material to make up the baby's heritage there was a moment of silence. Then Susan said: "You mean I'm not the one who caused the baby's retardation?"

"We can't always answer that question," Laura responded. "But we do know that both parents contribute a set of genes. When we are able to study the baby's chromosome makeup we will understand more about what happened."

A conversation such as this one between the Collinses and Laura Thompson may not seem terribly important to a person who has not had the frightening experience of parenting a defective child. But mothers who have lived a lifetime in anguish because they believed themselves personally responsible for having passed bad genes on to a child will appreciate the significance. A great deal of this agony can be eliminated if the parents learn very soon after such a birth that *both* parents are responsible for the way an infant is created.

Despite training and experience in helping people cope with illness, some health professionals frequently do not understand the emotional impact that the birth of a defective infant may have on parents. Some even think it is helpful to appeal to the better instincts of parents rather than to help them express their intense, usually negative, feelings. This approach actually does little more than anger parents, and leads them to believe in fact that no one can give them the help they need.

One father expressed his reaction this way:

I think obstetricians should play a much stronger role in discussing these situations with parents. If only our doctor had come and sat down with us to answer our questions and our fears. Instead, we were made to feel this was a situation which couldn't be handled by anyone. One feels that if the professionals can't handle it, then you can't either. I couldn't find anyone to get help from.

Even today, some genetic counseling still consists of pointing out to couples that much "moral" good can come from having had a defective child! Sometimes genetic counselors have even gone so far as to comment that "only special people" are chosen by God for such responsibility and that these parents should respond with love and acceptance of this "bad baby." Any failure on the part of the parents to have such glorious feelings, when they have been told that this is the "right" reaction to such a birth, will naturally horrify the parents and make them feel they are abnormal because of their inability to feel "good" about their defective child.

One couple who faced such a birth remembers their anger and fury that "it had to happen to us!" "Everyone around us," they are now able to report, "found these feelings of ours a burden and stayed away from us as much as possible." The wife added that she "absolutely rejected the baby. I couldn't cope with how this had happened to me."

"CONSPIRACY OF SILENCE"

Other parents of defective children tell tragic stories of how they themselves have been rejected upon their child's birth. Such parents feel they have been rejected by obstetricians, pediatricians, and even nurses, all of whom have seemed incapable of talking to them about what has happened.

A new mother said that she "knew in the delivery room that something was wrong. When I began to come out of the anesthesia everyone had left the room except for one little nurse standing by the delivery table. When I asked her 'what I had' she said, 'the doctor will tell you.' Then it began. Nobody wanted to talk to me."

This "conspiracy of silence" toward the parents of a defective baby often causes them to sense that they have done something "wrong." This, they tend to think, must be why they are being ignored by the professionals upon whom they so desperately depend. Many parents of babies with genetic diseases and birth defects report that it is sometimes months before they are able to realize what has happened to them as a result of this rejection by the medical staff. "It makes for very bitter feelings," one mother said. Few such mothers ever return to the obstetricians who were so incapable of providing the necessary emotional support in their time of great need. Some of these parents refuse to pay their medical bills to physicians who have been so insensitive.

This type of counseling—or lack of it—is inappropriate and certainly does not help families deal with their intense and usually negative feelings about the misfortune which produced a defective infant. Even for those families who are not conflicted about their wish to care for such babies at home, there is still a real need to offer them immediate help in understanding what went wrong with this particular pregnancy.

If a family can be helped to recognize that their negative feelings are entirely normal under the circumstances, it will allow them to relate to a counselor in a positive way. It will help them to look upon a genetic counselor as someone who can be trusted, and who may be able to help them manage their unfortunate situation. Because of their experience, counselors are often able to provide considerable information to families about community resources for training and caring for children with genetic diseases.

Parents, fraught with guilt and other strong emotions, must be told that their reactions to the birth of a genetically defective child are not disgraceful. Many couples will find comfort in groups consisting of parents who have had similar problem births. One mother said, after her genetically damaged baby was born: "I desperately wanted to meet other mothers who had the same experiences, but no one listened to me." A father of a Down syndrome child recently suggested a program in which parents who already have had the experience of producing affected children would visit new parents soon after the birth of a defective child.

It is a real tragedy today that parents who find themselves in the situation of having given birth to a child with a genetic defect are forced to "get hold of themselves" alone, in order to be able to ask for the help they so badly need. Someday, perhaps, the need will be recognized more readily by the professionals themselves, who will then be able to offer this help at once. Parent groups such as the one suggested by the father mentioned above have been formed in some parts of the country and can be of tremendous value.

FINDING THE GENETIC COUNSELOR

Many formulas have been developed to help prospective patients find a doctor or dentist of a particular type. Unfortunately not all these guidelines are applicable to finding a genetic counselor, at least not at the present time. The reason for this is that genetic counseling, as either a specialized field in itself or as a specialty of medicine, is so new that no professional boards have been established yet to help screen practitioners for their degree of knowledge and training in this field.

The matter is further complicated because the subject of human genetics is so complex that a single health care professional cannot really run a "solo" genetics practice without a considerable amount of help from other specialists, laboratories, diagnostic facilities, and many ancillary personnel such as social workers, public health nurses, and genetic associates.

If a family's physician suggests the need for genetic counseling, then it is possible that the physician can make a referral to a center that offers these services.

Many families who seek genetic counseling, however, do not go through a primary-care physician in the first place. While the reasons for this are not clear, we suspect that the physicians' unfamiliarity with the importance of genetic disease makes them unsympathetic to requests for such referrals. In such cases, the family may go directly to a genetics center that they already have heard about, or they may consult one of several voluntary health organizations which act as clearinghouses for genetic counseling services. One of these, the National Foundation–March of Dimes (see Appendix I for address) maintains a computerized listing of several hundred genetic counseling and diagnostic centers throughout the United States. A number of these are listed in Appendix II at the end of this book.

There has been a good deal of controversy as to whether the primary genetic counselor ought to be a physician with special training in human genetics and related fields, or a Ph.D. geneticist with special training in genetic counseling.

It is likely that genetic counseling will remain an interdisciplinary field, open to qualified physicians and Ph.D.'s, the best of whom will recognize their own limitations and will avail themselves of the consulting services of their colleagues with related expertise.

Many health insurance programs at present do not cover genetic counseling as such. However, the physical examination and diagnostic tests which may be a major part of the testing-counseling process very often *are* covered by health insurance under the heading of "diagnostic tests."

There is little doubt that as public demand increases, more and more health insurance policies will begin to pay for comprehensive genetic counseling services as well.

CHAPTER

5

YOU AND
YOUR DOCTOR

MOST ADULTS WHO ARE PLANNING TO HAVE CHILDREN want to be responsible with respect to both the family's size and its health.

Ideally, every general practitioner, internist, pediatrician, and obstetrician should be as aware of your genetic heritage as he or she is concerned for your general physical health. But even today information about genetics and inheritance is often a major gap in the knowledge of the average practicing physician. If this sounds alarming to you, it should. In 1975 the National Academy of Sciences surveyed 1,000 physicians in order to learn about their understanding and training in human genetics. The survey revealed that of all the pediatricians, obstetricians, and family practitioners polled, only one-half correctly answered questions about the frequency of genetic defects in the population.

The pediatricians scored the highest number of correct answers, with only 55.8 percent! The family physicians only scored 43.6 percent correct responses, in spite of the fact that this specialty field deals with a tremendous number of women in their childbearing years. Only 46.5 percent of the obstetricians surveyed considered it to be "extremely important" to detect potential or actual genetic disorders. This in spite of the fact that genetic diseases or their complications account for nearly 40 percent of all pediatric hospital admissions.

Many of the readers of this book will be—or are—receiving their medical care from the 50 percent of the physicians like those polled, whose understanding of genetics is woefully inadequate. So it is up to you to demand that responsible attention be paid to this important aspect of your health. Some young women already understand this and take matters into their own hands. Emily, for example, knew that her doctor's reasoning was wrong when he told her not to bother to come in for Tay Sachs disease testing because he "had never delivered a Tay Sachs infant." As Emily said, "I figured there could be a first time, so I'm getting the test."

In a textbook published in 1975, Edmond A. Murphy and Gary A. Chase, both prominent geneticists, admitted that it "would be difficult to find a field of science in which there is a greater failure of communication between the basic scientist and the practitioner," than in genetics.

QUESTION THE DOCTOR

It is primarily for this reason that it is so important for the couple planning a family to enter the obstetrician's office armed with the knowledge that their questions—and even their fears—are not necessarily unreasonable. As we have seen, such questions are actually so important that they may mean the difference between joy and sorrow as a parent. And the specific information in the hands of an interested and educated parent may in fact be "news" to the doctor.

Don't be concerned with what the doctor thinks about you if you come armed with pages of questions written out. The physician may grimace when he sees your notes, but more than one doctor has told us that he much prefers intelligent and informed patients to those who come totally unaware of their condition.

Remember that, as the "consumer," you are engaging the physician to do a job for you—in the case of an expectant couple, the doctor is consulted to advise the parents and to provide them with help of many kinds until the desired goals are reached as closely as possible. These goals, of course, are for a healthy baby, a healthy mother, a healthy family.

Questions parents have usually concern their own physical health and how it may relate to their children's well-being. Although much has been written about the dangers of drugs and X rays, most parents today are unclear about the extent of such danger and are often very worried. Prospective parents *should* be concerned about their family's medical history and attempt to discover the implications for their offspring of specific illnesses which may run in their family. In addition to questions about medical history, many parents want to know their doctor's views on the use of anesthesia during childbirth and how he or she will act if the baby has a physical or mental defect that is obvious at birth.

If the physician you choose refuses to spend enough time with you to answer to your satisfaction all your questions, then there is a good chance that you have chosen the wrong physician for you. If you leave the doctor's office with unanswered questions, you have not received the full treatment for which you—or your health insurance—have paid.

You should also keep in mind the possibility that a doctor who abruptly dismisses your questions as unimportant or insignificant may be a physician who is not knowledgeable about a particular issue. It was a wise physician who once observed that even the simplest question posed by a patient was actually a very important question if it was troubling the patient enough to ask it.

Take, for instance, the poignant story of the forty-year-old pregnant woman who, early in her pregnancy, asked her obstetrician if there was a great risk in pregnancy at her age. She was asking, she said, because she had once read in a woman's magazine about a test for older pregnant women.

The physician reassured the woman, and told her there was "nothing to worry about. After all, I have never delivered a mongoloid baby in my twenty-three years of obstetric practice."

In spite of this the woman was not reassured, and she traveled many miles to seek proper advice. Unfortunately, by the time she received it she was already twenty-two weeks pregnant and it was too late for her to undergo amniocentesis which would, indeed, have revealed that she was among the one in every 3,000 women in the United States who would bear a child with Down syndrome that year. At age forty, however, this woman's risk was not one in 3,000, but one in 80, a risk that most forty-year-old women feel is high enough to warrant the proper tests to determine whether there may be problems with their pregnancies.

How can we explain the obstetrician who fails to offer such important advice to pregnant women older than age thirty-five?—all of whom should be urged to undergo amniocentesis, according to all leading geneticists. There is no excuse. Physicians are professionally obligated to discuss prenatal diagnosis with all of their "older" pregnant patients, as well as others who may be at risk. Realistically, it is every woman's right to choose or to decline this, or any other medical procedure. But whatever she ultimately decides upon, it is essential that she understand what the risks are at her age, and that she make her decision with the advice of her physician. It is *not* the physician's job to tell the patient what to do.

One can only suspect that an obstetrician such as the one discussed earlier, who has delivered "thousands of babies," begins to believe that it is he—not the genes—who ultimately determines the outcome of pregnancy.

THE GENETIC CONNECTION

It is also important to add at this point that only obstetricians who have been trained during the past fifteen years have been taught human genetics in medical school. So if your obstetrician was trained before that time, it is quite possible that he honestly thinks you don't have to worry about the genetic risks we have discussed. The literature is full of sad stories about couples who have been told that they have "nothing to worry about," but who turn out to be *the one* in those "one-in-a-million" statistics we so often hear about.

How should the physician concern himself or herself with your genetic risk? Many women consult a gynecologist long before they begin to plan their families. The gynecologist, who often becomes the woman's obstetrician—or, for that matter, any other primary-care physician—should take a family history (pedigree) at the same time as the initial routine medical history is being taken, on the patient's first visit.

THE HISTORY IS THE KEY

A detailed family history—called the pedigree—seeks to determine what illnesses have commonly occurred in one's family for at least as far back as one generation and preferably for three generations and, most important, what the family's experience has been with childbirth. A complete pedigree should also include a discussion about brothers and sisters of both of the prospective parents, and their reproductive experiences.

The importance of such questioning is not at all difficult to illustrate. One physician tells of an attractive young woman in her thirties who was profoundly afraid of marrying and having children for fear "they will be retarded just like everyone else in my family." At least one sibling, several cousins, and other relatives of this young woman were mentally retarded. She had decided for herself that this was a hereditary defect that she carried and had absolutely convinced herself she would never have children, and thus she avoided meaningful relationships with men. Upon study of a tissue sample from this woman, however, physicians were able to assure her that she carried no chromosomal abnormalities that would result in hereditary mental retardation.

A second example of the value of discussing the family history with your physician can be seen clearly by looking at a couple in which the husband's brother has cystic fibrosis. If neither the husband nor wife in question is aware that cystic fibrosis is a hereditary disease, they may never tell the doctor about the husband's brother. If the couple's physician fails to question them and elicit this information while taking a family history, the couple may never know that:

1 / Perfectly healthy individuals can carry the gene for cystic fibrosis. In fact, it is carried by one in twenty white individuals.

2 / The husband has an even greater chance of carrying the CF gene because his brother has the disease.

3 / If the wife is also a carrier, each time they bear a child there will be a 25-percent chance that the child will have cystic fibrosis disease.

About 1 in every 400 white couples are carriers of cystic fibrosis (that is, both the man and the woman are carriers of the cystic fibrosis gene). Therefore the risk of bearing a child with cystic fibrosis is not such a remote possibility and if one's brother has cystic fibrosis the possibility is much higher.

Thus it is vital for individuals and their physicians to know what harmful genes each person, or his or her mate, may carry. In the case of cystic fibrosis, prenatal diagnosis is not yet able to pick out fetuses which carry this gene. Some might argue, therefore, that knowledge of a family history of this disease is irrelevant, since nothing can be done about it at the present time. It is probable, however, that most prospective parents would want to know about potential risks for bearing a child with a disease such as cystic fibrosis. It is true that many couples would go ahead and "take the chance" on having a healthy child. On the other hand, some couples might refrain from having children altogether, preferring to remain childless, to adopt, or to have a child by artificial insemination.

The ethnic heritage of both members of a couple is another important area that should be covered in a comprehensive family history. Questions about this aspect of your heritage may help to determine whether you are at risk for having children with conditions such as Tay Sachs disease, thalassemia, or sickle-cell anemia, to name just a few of the diseases associated with specific ethnic groups. Since many people aren't aware of which diseases may be inherited, it is important for your doctor to ascertain whether any disease specific to your ethnic group has occurred in your family. This kind of information can serve as an important diagnostic tool for the physician.

THE NEXT STEP IS UP TO YOU

If an individual or a couple is found to be at risk for any of the known genetically determined diseases, they will doubtlessly be quite alarmed, and properly so. Neither the parent nor the physician should ignore this legitimate concern. Statistics of the "one-in-a-million" variety may be reassuring in a textbook, but when they refer to your future as a parent there is no way to diminish your anxiety except through a careful evaluation of the genetic condition for which you may be at risk.

As one parent observed, "Facts and figures are important. But feelings are more important."

Once an expert evaluation has been made of the various aspects of your liability toward a particular genetic disease, the next step is up to you. You and your mate should be prepared to take the responsibility for making the decisions that will affect your future and the future of your children. Of course you will want to rely on the experts for guidance and information. The importance of accurate diagnosis of any genetic problem cannot be stressed too much.

Many individuals choose to seek genetic counseling before they start their families. This kind of planning gives a couple freedom from the pressure of time associated with needing an amniocentesis by the seventeenth week of pregnancy, for example, and offers time for the couple to come to terms with the risk both emotionally and medically. However, there is no test that can guarantee a couple that their children will be perfect in every respect.

Faced with the risk of bearing a genetically diseased child, you may want to talk to the experts who can explain the long-range aspects of the particular disease, should it occur. You may need some psychological counseling to help you cope with the strain that the discovery of the "bad genes" will inevitably place on your marriage. Both of you are only deceiving yourselves if you do not recognize the fact that any possibility of genetic imperfection may rock the foundations of even the most secure relationship.

FINDING THE RIGHT DOCTOR

Many prospective mothers will want to choose a physician who will regard their physical health as the first priority. It is important for these women to ask their physician about his or her opinions regarding the priorities of childbirth and about any religious beliefs that might influence them. Physicians have every right to their own religious and moral beliefs, but patients have an equally strong right to feel confident that their physician shares their opinion as to which is the primary concern, the mother or the fetus, should the need to make that decision arise.

It is equally important for mothers who believe the fetus should be saved at all costs to communicate this belief to their physician. Some mothers are determined to do everything within their power to produce only healthy children. For such a woman it would be important to determine whether her obstetrician had any religious or ethical values which might interfere with this goal.

Remember that 3 to 5 percent of the births in America will result in children with a significant birth defect. It is important that when a known risk such as this is present, prospective parents understand the full range of possible problems associated with the condition.

This means that the parents will want to talk to an internist, a pediatrician, or a family doctor who is frank in telling them what the child's physical and mental potential may be.

A sensitive physician will not leave parents who have given birth to a child with a genetic disease uninformed about the situation. Unfortunately, however, not all physicians behave so responsibly. One man recalled how he tried for seven hours to reach the pediatrician, who had told the man's wife after the father had left the hospital that their child had been born with Down syndrome. This father had been in the delivery room throughout his wife's four-hour labor, but as soon as the delivery was completed, the obstetrician rushed out of the hospital without a word to the parents.

Later the parents realized that the physician was "running away from us." Other obstetricians, who feel strongly that parents should be given a much more positive sense about what has happened, do not run away from parents in distress. Unfortunately some of the caring physicians do not properly inform themselves about the heritability of the newborn's condition. One such obstetrician who delivered a child suffering from anencephaly—a severe brain defect with a 3- to 5-percent chance of recurring—told his patient that it was "nothing to worry about. You'll get pregnant again immediately and you won't even remember this bad experience."

Although many families have an enormous capacity to deal with physical problems in a child, other families are overwhelmed by the same situation. It is impossible to speculate on anyone's capacity in this connection, or on the burden that a given condition may place upon a specific family physically, economically, or psychologically. But once a husband and wife are made aware by the genetic counseling team of the various options available to them as parents, they must decide for themselves how they will handle the situation. If a first child is born with a genetic disease, the stresses will obviously be very different than if there are already three healthy children in the family, for example.

THE DOCTOR'S RESPONSIBILITIES

In addition to the moral and professional responsibilities of a physician to fully discuss potential genetic problems with his patients, there are also legal obligations. While it is true that genetics and genetic counseling are relatively new fields, physicians have, nevertheless, already been held responsible by several courts for failing to impart such information to prospective parents.

Philip Reilly, an attorney at the Medical Genetics

Center at the University of Texas Graduate School of Biomedical Sciences at Houston, and Dr. Aubrey Milunsky, a geneticist from Harvard Medical School, wrote in the *American Journal of Law and Medicine* that

> Ignorance by the physician of such a major advance [as genetic counseling and prenatal diagnosis], which is now a part of established medical practice, cannot be condoned. Hence, failure by the physician to inform a pregnant woman that she is at risk for having offspring with a certain genetic disease could expose him to legal liability.

The doctor and the lawyer go on to say that physicians surely have the right to their own religious beliefs, and if they choose not to involve themselves in amniocentesis or prenatal genetic studies that is their prerogative. But they must be willing to refer patients to physicians who are both competent and willing to provide these services.

> Errors both of omission and commission would make the physician culpable in the new practice of prenatal genetic diagnosis. The deliberate intent or carelessness of the physician manifest in his or her failure to inform such a patient that there is a need for an amniocentesis and prenatal studies invites suit.

In a 1976 article in the *Journal of Legal Medicine,* a father-son, doctor-lawyer team of Dr. Henry Lynch and Patrick Lynch talked about possible genetic links of certain types of cancers. Their conclusions, however, are relevant to all aspects of inherited disease.

> In those cases where such risk information can be utilized effectively in cancer control and prevention, patients necessarily will come to expect their physicians to under-

stand more adequately genetic risk information and act on it when treating themselves and other family members. It is hoped that these expectations will not be frustrated, for malpractice litigation generally arises where legitimate patient expectations are not met. . . . Taking a thorough family history and comprehending its implications should not be regarded simply as another defensive safeguard to avoid liability, but as a valuable diagnostic tool.

Along the same lines, physicians also have the responsibility to inform their patients of carrier detection tests for genetic diseases such as Tay Sachs disease or sickle-cell anemia, wherever they are relevant.

Up to this point we have mainly discussed the expectations consumers can rightfully have of physicians who counsel them before they have children. Now we turn to the more difficult question of what kind of medical attention you should seek if you bear a child with a genetic disease or other birth defect.

The story of June and Stan Greenhouse illustrates the problem. They had two healthy children when their third child was born with spina bifida, a crippling and sometimes fatal spinal cord defect. The child was born at a community hospital that did not have facilities to care for such serious birth defects, so the child was transferred to a large medical center several hours after birth. The baby's "open spine" meant that a number of surgical operations would be necessary, but even with this help the child might never be able to walk or to have proper control of either his bowel or bladder.

As soon as their baby was born the Greenhouses were told that he was seriously ill and had to be transferred to a special care nursery.

"Naturally we were too upset to ask many questions," Stan later recalled.

June explained that "We made all the necessary arrangements and Stan went to the second hospital when the baby was admitted. They asked Stan to sign several papers which he didn't understand, partly because he was very nervous and partly because the doctor didn't explain what would be done to the baby—just that they had to operate quickly."

The next day Stan met with the surgeon, who told him that the baby had many problems and that several more operations would be required. By this time Stan had become calmer and more rational and he asked the doctor two questions: Would the baby ever be normal? What would happen if they didn't operate?

To the first question the surgeon replied "probably not," and to the second question he gave a very evasive reply.

Stan learned, however, that withholding further treatment meant the baby would die, although no one could predict how long this would take.

"We were astonished that it had taken three days for the doctors to give us the whole story and we wondered if they would have told us anything like this if we hadn't asked such direct questions," June said later.

WHAT TO ASK THE DOCTOR

While it may seem obvious to expect that the parents would be given a complete picture of their baby's problem, the prospects for the future, and the suspected reasons for any abnormality, it is probably clear to you by this time that medical care in the area of birth defects may be less than ideal. Such information may not always be readily offered by your physician, and you may need to ask for additional detailed information about your child's problems and potential. Parents who feel they cannot bring their affected children home certainly need considerable guidance as to what alternatives are available. Private care, institutional care, and foster care are some of the possibilities. In addition, parents will want to know, for example:

1 / Is the condition a known hereditary disease?

2 / What is the likely prognosis? What is the child's potential?

3 / Is there any treatment or cure?

4 / Is extended hospitalization likely to be necessary, and if so, will financial help be available from the government or from private organizations?

5 / What is the possibility that any subsequent children will suffer the same abnormality?

6 / Is prenatal diagnosis available for this disorder in future pregnancies?

7 / Can other family members be tested to see if they are carriers of the disorder?

8 / What is the risk that normal siblings and other family members will have problems with their children?

Both you and your partner should insist that you be given this information *together* to insure that each of you receive the same facts and thus avoid confusion or misinterpretation. It is also vital for each of you to be present at this time to help the other partner emotionally.

Some parents will feel that it is better for them to

bear the burden of the defective child alone, and they will try to shield their partners from the specifics of the condition. But experience has shown that families do not really have the capacity to keep secrets such as these. Partners eventually will learn the facts, often more painfully than if they had been shared initially.

Some weeks after delivery of your child, when the genetic studies are completed, you will meet with the geneticist. His or her diagnosis will probably be discussed with you in person and subsequently sent to you in writing. This written record is important to keep for future reference, and you should ask to have it if it is not provided automatically.

If your newborn suffers from one of the more severe physical birth defects, the option or necessity of surgery may be an issue for immediate concern. Every hospital and every physician will handle this kind of situation in their own ways. But what is often not made perfectly clear to parents at this time is that the decision whether to operate on a child should be theirs to make.

DIFFICULT DECISIONS

Ideally, the pediatrician and the surgeon will discuss the situation with you in a detailed manner, allowing you to consider all of the various options and possibilities.

You will be under tremendous stress at the time, and there will be a number of factors at play about which you may be unaware. On the one hand, for example, the doctors are under great pressure to defend each of their medical actions—or lack of action—in view of the continuing malpractice crisis. In addition, the entire professional life of the physician is traditionally devoted to saving lives. For the most part, physicians are single-minded in this devotion, and they usually allow little consideration of other factors which might influence the medical options open to them. Most of the other health professionals, such as nurses, will share similar attitudes and goals, since it is the physician who sets the tone for the entire medical team. In this regard, then, it is important for you to remember that the medical attitude is one of action (i.e., treatment). Successful therapy, of course, is always the goal, but even medical treatments with limited chances of success, or little value, are preferred over inaction by many physicians. Some physicians, however, are beginning to ask themselves and their colleagues whether a lifesaving procedure *should* be carried out, rather than *can* such a procedure be accomplished.

In the case of children with severe birth defects where the quality of life that is possible is far from ideal, it is essential that parents and physicians *together* make the decision whether massive efforts to maintain life should be continued or whether such an infant should be allowed to die. Now that people in our society are beginning to openly discuss the option of not maintaining the life of severely defective newborn babies, much has been said about the "cruelty and pain" of withdrawing life support.

Public discussion of the option of not maintaining the life of severely defective newborns is a development of the 1970s. In years past, this was one of the "taboo" topics.

By 1974, however, the question had reached the stage at which it could even be discussed in a daily newspaper. The following letter was written by a prospective father from Denver, to a newspaper health columnist:

> You may think this is a cruel thing to ask, but my wife and I are planning to have our first child in a year or so. But if, by a rare chance, the baby turns out to be born with severe physical or brain defects we don't want him or her to have to live through even a year of life with the agony. Our problem is that we want to make sure that the doctor who delivers our baby feels the same way we do. We don't want him to be a hero and save a baby that is destined to misery. How can we be sure we get a doctor that thinks this way?

The only way to answer a question such as this is to once again stress the word "communication"—that is, open and frank communication between patient and doctor. In spite of what the prospective father thinks, his question is not "cruel," nor even unusual. Indeed, whether they admit it or not, all parents-to-be are faced with similar fears and concerns. The good doctor understands such emotions, and helps patients cope with them.

LETTING BABIES DIE

Several years ago, an article appeared in the *New England Journal of Medicine,* written by two physicians associated with the Yale-New Haven Hospital. The detailed article discussed forty-three severely deformed infants who had been allowed to die during a two-year period which the doctors had studied.

"They were severely malformed children who had an extremely bleak outlook and treatment was withheld. Instead of saying the infants were allowed to die, you ought to say we didn't fight to prolong their lives," said pediatrician Raymond Duff, one of the authors.

One must realize, however, that the real difficulty in such a situation is determining that a particular defect will really mean a few years of misery and then an inevitable early death. Sometimes the situation is very clear, but other times it is not an easy decision to make.

When the article in the *New England Journal* was reported in the daily press, many people were outraged that these events took place at all. But doctors explain that this practice is really not new.

Allowing hopelessly ill patients to die is "accepted medical practice," at many hospitals, commented Dr. Lawrence K. Pickett, chief of staff at the Yale-New Haven Hospital.

What was new at the time of the public furor, however, and continues to be so, is the fact that these topics are now being openly discussed. "I think it's a good thing to get this out and discuss it, because it's a common denominator at every nursery in the country," Dr. Pickett said.

Even according to major religious doctrine this practice is not without some support. In 1958, Pope Pius XII said that if a person's life is ebbing hopelessly, doctors may cease their efforts, thus "to permit the patient, already virtually dead, to pass on in peace." He noted also that heroic measures are not indicated in hopeless situations.

In 1961, Britain's chief Rabbi Immanuel Jakobovits stated that "Jewish law sanctions the withdrawal of any factor—whether extraneous to the patient himself or not—which may artificially delay his demise in the final phase."

Surely it is hopeless to perform agonizing and extensive operations on a newborn infant who, even if all the surgery is successful, will at best be crippled, deformed, and profoundly retarded.

In spite of all the dialogue that has gone on in this area over the past several years, some health professionals and some hospital administrators will try to make parents feel that they are attempting to "murder" their own child when they raise the possibility of not continuing heroic treatment in drastic cases. One such couple was told that if they refused surgical consent, their baby would be put in a corner of the nursery to "starve to death." How can a parent rationally deal with this kind of advice? Is this the kind of medical guidance that is really designed to help parents make an informed choice? Or is it advice that comes from a narrow-minded professional who is trying to impose his or her own values on a parent?

Experience has shown that families who agree to medical care under duress by insistent physicians or hospital administrators remain resentful and conflicted over the result for the rest of their lives.

Given the proper opportunity and guidance, it is entirely possible that parents will reach the same decision advocated by the professional, but at least it will have been their own decision, and it will have been achieved through a process of dignity and of respect for their rights as parents. It is far more humane for physicians to recognize openly the conflicts parents will inevitably be confronted with during such crises. They must honestly discuss the medical possibilities and consequences, including the fact that in many newborn crises, the infant will die a natural death if treatment is withheld.

For those parents who will have to deal with these very difficult decisions in the future there is hope, for an increasing number of health professionals are now viewing these problems of childbirth with greater awareness of the need for parents to share in the decision making. Not only does this sharing of responsibility make good sense, but it relieves physicians of the burden of having to be omnipotent, a role no human being can possibly hope to fulfill.

In some intensive care nurseries, each family is given all the staff support possible to reach a decision that is comfortable for them. When this involves allowing an infant to die, those parents who wish to be involved are helped to care for the infant and even to hold it as it dies. Nurseries which are able to offer this kind of total family care, while rare, recognize the wishes of such parents as positive acts of responsibility and, as such, worthy of total support. Health professionals who serve in such settings are generally endowed with a nonjudgmental kind of professionalism which allows them to focus primarily on the family in crisis.

CHAPTER

6

THE
PARENTHOOD
MYSTIQUE

IN SPITE OF THE REMARKABLE ADVANCES IN BIOLOGY AND medicine that have led to the freedom to make choices about family planning, prospective parents still pay surprisingly little attention to the complexities of producing the three million babies who are born every year in the United States. Of those three million, about 16,000 will have some form of genetic abnormality.

Statistics? Yes. But when one woman was told of a diagnosed defect in the child she was carrying, she observed, "You spend all your life looking at pictures of pretty babies and their mothers and thinking that will be you. It's pretty gruesome when you are the one who is different."

Responsibility and concern for one's own health should go hand in hand with concern over the health of one's prospective children. However, even in a contemporary book such as the best-selling *Our Bodies, Ourselves,* which captured the interest of so many young women, only half a page is devoted to the potential genetic problems of pregnancy.

THE PARENTHOOD MYSTIQUE

Most people accept the age-old parental role of perpetuating civilization from one generation to the next by bringing children into the world. Since biblical times pregnancy has been considered woman's destiny as well as her fulfillment. Poets have written about the idea expressed by a mother who said, "Becoming a mother, I really felt legitimate as a person."

Historian Lois Banner expressed the idea this way: "A man, whether bachelor or father, widower or gentleman, is primarily a man. A woman, on the other hand, is defined by the role she plays." Man's drive toward parenthood is often thought to be more in the form of an instinct for survival. Whatever the true meaning of parenthood, we know that bearing children is an event of enormous significance to both men and women. In fact, part of the marriage dream for most couples—indeed a kind of unspoken marriage contract—consists of the wish to have children. The expectation, of course, is that those children will be healthy, and about 96 percent of all children born in the world today are healthy.

On the other hand, the inability to become a parent or to produce a normal child is deeply disturbing to those women and men who have had this experience.

Contracts generally imply that the two parties involved share the commitment and responsibility for successfully completing the matter at hand. When a portion of a contract—either formal or informal—is not fulfilled, the parties to the contract may experience a sense of anger that their partner has not fulfilled his or her share of the bargain. This anger may well occur when an imperfect baby is born.

Women are emotionally more susceptible to blame in the accidents of childbearing because of their traditional and physical role as childbearers. It is clear, however, that both parents share equally in the genetic as well as the emotional burdens of this marital role.

The experiences of one couple in their late twenties, who gave birth to their first child after two years of marriage, illustrates some of these conflicts.

Alice and her husband, Tom, were members of a large family in New York City. The couple expected to have many healthy children, just as each of their own parents had. Instead, their first child was a little girl who was diagnosed as suffering from Down syndrome.

Both Alice and Tom, who is a police officer, knew what retarded children were like. Tom, in fact, had been involved in a police force program to raise funds for recreational facilities for retarded youngsters. But now, after having dreamed about becoming parents, their promises to each other had failed. Even though neither Tom nor Alice was at "fault"—at least in a way they were able to control—their baby was not normal and never would be.

THE GENETIC CONNECTION

For some men, fatherhood proclaims virility. Some men report the experience of becoming a father is "like a high, a dazed, off-the-ground, feeling-ten-feet-tall experience." New fathers have described themselves as feeling "proud, bigger, older."

THE "GOOD GENE" MYTH

Similarly, both men and women have a deep-seated need to believe that they possess "good genes." Women who feel they have so-called "bad genes" often refer to themselves as "imperfect, inferior, unfeminine, inadequate." Knowledge of the presence of less-than-perfect genes seems to implicate the quality of one's sexuality. Parenthood itself is often seen as the fulfillment of one's sexual being, though there is no basis in reality—i.e., biology—for such feelings. Nevertheless, myths are powerful forces that do not die easily.

The drive to accomplish the "perfect" experience of parenting a healthy child is so strong in some people that one father who had already sired two severely defective children told of his intention to go on having children until he and his wife "get a good one."

Another thirty-two-year-old father of three children had just been diagnosed as having a progressive, inherited neurological disease. Since the disease does not usually manifest itself until later in life, there was a 50-percent chance that each of his present children had already inherited the gene, and would later suffer its ill effects. This father seems to exemplify the need of many men and women to "prove" themselves in the genetic sense. In spite of the fact that he already had sired three children before his heritable condition was discovered, he insisted upon continuing to have children, and stressed his idea that there was no substitute for life, however imperfect that life might be.

For this man to say to himself and to his immediate world that he should father no more children would have been like admitting he was no longer manly, since fatherhood for him symbolized his masculinity.

Someday there will be a prenatal test available to determine if such people who carry these defective genes have passed them on to their offspring. As of this moment, however, certain genetic diseases which do not develop until mid-life cannot be predicted before their symptoms appear. We know only that this young man, and others like him, will have a 50-percent chance of passing to each of his children the same genetic defect that he carries within his body.

Pregnancy has sometimes been described as a "normal illness." This implies that the whole process of pregnancy is a time of both physical and emotional stress—and growth—for a woman. Many women—and men, too—still see motherhood as the true destiny of women. It is easy to understand that the emotions aroused by this important event in one's life are powerful, sometimes overwhelming. At times of crisis one's whole being is under stress. Those individuals who have had trouble facing simple life problems may, therefore, have even more difficulty with major changes in life, such as parenthood.

A strong and supportive relationship with one's own parents can often help a couple through the "crisis of pregnancy." However, when relations with parents are strained, it may place even more strain on one's ability to handle pregnancy and childbirth, particularly if things do not go perfectly. As one experienced mother observed, "Mothers have to help daughters a lot when bad babies are born."

Alice and Tom, the couple we discussed earlier, whose first child was born with Down syndrome, were at first unable to talk about their defective child and the sense of loss each of them felt at not having a normal child. They each tried to deny how serious the condition was. When they were eventually referred to a specialty clinic with their baby, each repeated what they remembered the pediatrician had said: "The chances are very good that there is nothing wrong with the baby."

Their tense behavior, however, belied their outward calm. Denial is an important mechanism that most people use to defend themselves against painful realities. In this situation, however, by not sharing their disappointment verbally with each other, Alice and Tom also denied themselves the benefit of the emotional support each badly needed. Perhaps their anger at one another for failing to fulfill their marriage contract made this impossible. But experience with families who have had defective children has made it clear that the first step in coping with a family crisis of this magnitude should be the sharing and recognition of the grief that parents always feel at such an event.

THE MARRIAGE DREAM

Let us now consider the emotional impact of marriage and reproduction. What actually happens mentally to the woman who falls in love, marries, and has children?

Theoretically she is in love with her sexual partner and as a by-product of this physical love she becomes pregnant. Thus the fetus growing within her in many ways represents both a biological and psychological part of herself. This foreign body, as it were, representing her love for her mate, merges with her and actually becomes a part of her own body. Eventually a woman begins to think of this other self as separate from herself, but this only occurs as the pregnancy progresses. In the meantime, however, the woman and her mate have actually fused, both emotionally and biologically, into a foreign object which, at the same time, is actually part of the woman herself.

If the fetus happens to be defective, then it is not difficult to understand a mother's sense of personal inadequacy, for she experiences it not only as a defective baby but as a defective part of herself. Thus, to many women, delivering a "good" baby—that is, a healthy one—really means that they are "good" mothers. If the baby is not "good" in these terms it can be a psychological disaster for the mother. Childbirth represents such a vulnerable time in a woman's life that an added blow of this nature can seriously weaken a woman's self-image.

One woman, for example, on learning that she carried a defective gene and that there was a 50-percent chance she had passed it on to her children, reacted by saying, "I felt I had to make myself whole again . . . something is wrong with me and I am wide open and hurting."

THE GENETIC CONNECTION

For many people, any public affirmation that they may be less than perfect—that they have bad genes, for example—is an embarrassment and a humiliation.

It is obvious, however, that most people don't go around describing themselves in these terms, so such feelings of inadequacy are usually expressed as depression and deep sadness for the defective child and its future. Our society's attachment to the "stiff upper lip" philosophy, which implies that to suffer is noble, makes it very difficult for parents to openly discuss with one another and their families the distress they are experiencing in such circumstances.

One mother said, for example, "If God wanted me to have a defective child, He will help me take care of it."

Many of the technologies described in this book will make it possible for parents to take important steps toward insuring that their children will be healthy. But for some parents this will not be possible. Those parents who do not have a genetically healthy child must understand how important it is to *communicate*.

Talk to each other! Do not assume that the pain and anguish you are feeling are unique to you. *Mothers*, do not imagine that your baby's father is not suffering just as you are. Remember, this man may be feeling that he's less of a man because the baby is imperfect, just as you probably feel somewhat imperfect as a woman. *Fathers*, you must help the mother express her grief over having lost the perfect baby she was expecting. You must help her realize that you do not think she is any less of a woman because your baby is less than perfect. You have produced this imperfect child *together*, but it was biology, not destiny, that determined this event.

EXPECT HOSTILE FEELINGS

Parents should also understand that they may harbor some very hostile feelings toward their defective child as well as toward each other. Since parents are supposed to love their children, according to our traditional heritage, such feelings of antipathy toward the defective child will tear at the deepest parental emotions.

"When I saw that there was something wrong with my baby, and I knew it would just never be normal and all that we wished for, I just wished she was dead," recalled one mother, who added, "Of course I couldn't say it to anyone. And then I realized that I must be one sick woman to wish that my own child was dead."

The fact is that as long as individuals do not become obsessive about such feelings, they are perfectly normal ones for the parents of a defective child to experience. Even under more normal circumstances some parents will occasionally wish that their baby had never been born. This wish is understandable, since even a healthy, normal baby is initially an intruder into what was formerly a very different kind of relationship. Siblings, too, will often harbor negative feelings, and they occasionally will make quiet wishes to themselves that they could once again become an "only child."

Profound guilt feelings also may arise among parents or siblings if a new baby—healthy or sick—does die.

((131))

Under such circumstances it must be stressed that it was some kind of a physical disease that led to the baby's death, and not the wishes of the parents or siblings. Wishes of this nature *cannot kill,* but the guilt feelings they arouse *can* have a serious effect.

In our society, great value is placed on being a good parent. Parents who have borne genetically defective children often think this is the result of something bad they have done during the pregnancy. Understanding how genes predict the type of fetus to be born helps us to understand reproduction rationally and to know that it is our genes, and not our behavior, that will determine the result.

Emotionally, however, some women will continue to believe that there is a connection between their attitudes and their genes. One mother who gave birth to a child with malformed shoulders and short arms sincerely believed this was due to an argument she had with her mother-in-law when she was three months pregnant. At the time of the argument the mother-in-law became incensed and shook the pregnant mother by the shoulders in an abusive way. Although she was not physically hurt, this young mother was convinced that her son's deformity was a direct consequence of this episode—a result of her bad relationship with the in-laws she disliked.

BIRTH DEFECT MYTHS AND FACTS

There are hundreds of misconceptions about the causes of birth defects. Some of the myths, for example, state that a personal indiscretion, frequent intercourse during pregnancy, or exposure to the sight of a malformed child can result in defective births. Not true.

Some birth defects, however, may not be hereditary —that is, caused by the genes. Instead they are the result of accidents or mutations caused by environmental factors at the time of conception, or even earlier.

Much is not understood about this process, but the fact is that the genetic makeup of the egg and the sperm are determined before fertilization, in other words, *before* intercourse ever takes place. Many prospective parents do not realize, however, that there are certain harmful activities in which they can indulge before pregnancy occurs that will affect the genetic makeup of their reproductive cells. Especially noteworthy is that both males and females should avoid heavy doses of radiation as well as any drug abuse at least 60 to 90 days before conception.

There is also *very strong* evidence that outside influences can have an important effect on cell development after the egg and sperm have united. Some infections, such as syphilis, and the use of certain drugs can cause severe malformations of the fetus, especially if the woman is exposed to these outside agents during the first three months of pregnancy. Thus, women in their childbearing years must be particularly careful about the drugs they use—prescription or nonprescription—or the X rays they submit to, because of the possibility they may unknowingly be pregnant and may subject their future child to these teratogens—agents which can cause a malformed child if taken after conception and up to the fourth month of pregnancy.

Medical science is learning much more about the exact stage in human development at which these substances can be harmful, but until such research is perfected the safest course is to guard against exposure to all potentially harmful agents during pregnancy.

Although the defects an infant may suffer from exposure to the dangerous environmental factors known as teratogens can be similar to an inherited or genetic defect, there is a difference which is crucial to the family. Birth defects caused by teratogens are *not* passed along from parent to child or generation to generation. This means that the diagnosis of a defect caused by one of these agents—a diagnosis that may not be easy to make—frees a couple from the pressure of the possibility that they might pass the same defect on to subsequent children.

There are hundreds of teratogens listed in a recent publication. The list includes drugs such as the anticonvulsant Dilantin (diphenylhydantoin), several anticancer drugs, tranquilizers, and certain vitamins; environmental factors such as cigarette-smoking and exposure to X rays; and viral agents such as rubella (German measles). Many physicians order pregnant women to avoid drugs of *all kinds*—even aspirin—during their first three months of pregnancy. It is very important that a woman seek medical care early in every pregnancy in order to help avoid such exposures, or to take the necessary steps, such as prenatal diagnosis, if she has already been exposed to such risks.

CHAPTER

7

HOW
THE FAMILY
COPES

IN FAMILIES WHERE GENETIC DISEASE IS PRESENT, EVERY aspect of family life may be affected. A discussion of some of these potential problems may help to alleviate their development in certain affected families. For discussion purposes only, we have covered each family member separately. In reality, of course, one family member's reactions cannot be considered apart from those of the family as a whole.

THE MOTHER

The special and exclusive relationship between women and children is one reason why mothers are particularly vulnerable emotionally when something goes wrong in childbirth. Since our culture often expects women to carry out the duties of motherhood more than it expects fathers to discharge the duties of fatherhood, women frequently assume they have a greater biological responsibility for their children. This unequal and unbalanced division of responsibility quite naturally leads to the assumption by uninformed parents that mothers are the major determinants of their infant's health.

A young mother, reflecting on the birth of her defective child, observed:

> I wanted to believe I could cope with this tragedy myself and although I was in despair I kept telling everyone I was doing fine. It was not easy to approach me. I was often curt, remote, and too proud. But actually I didn't feel I deserved help. I had been delivered of a baby who was going to die. I felt I had failed everyone I cared about. I was not worthy of help, nor a new dress, nor a dinner out. When I did pull myself together and go out I would often be overcome by such sorrow as I have never experienced before or since. It is this overwhelming feeling of inadequacy that I think is so important to overcome. Perhaps it is based on the attitude that anyone can have babies, but not everyone can have babies who are healthy. Still, this inability is not a sign of worthlessness and we must help mothers of bad babies to go through the experience and then continue to live useful and contented lives.

Another woman reported upon learning that she was a carrier of a genetic disease that her stress was constant and confusing and that:

> . . . in a strange way I had to make myself whole again. I wondered if I would go through the rest of my life thinking of this constantly. . . . Eventually I came to

the realization that the heart of my emotional reaction involved the feeling of my being defective in some way. . . . I could begin to think and speak about being a carrier without distress only when I was able to view myself positively again.

Women who have aborted children also may suffer intense feelings of being less feminine and less maternal. This reaction, in turn, may lead to a sense of unworthiness and guilt, and perhaps to a feeling that they have destroyed something of themselves. This shame about oneself is usually heightened by the prevailing social attitudes toward the abortion procedure itself.

Although women who abort a fetus because it is known to be genetically defective *may* not suffer the same degree of shame, it is worth noting that similar reactions of guilt often result from abortion for whatever reason. When the pregnancy was a desired one, an abortion due to a defective fetus may even be more traumatic. Most women can be greatly helped by an opportunity to discuss these feelings with a trained counselor. Reactions of such intensity need to be resolved by every woman before she can return to a state of emotional health and equilibrium.

Mothers who have problem births are almost universally advised to become pregnant again as soon as possible. The physicians who give this kind of advice seem to believe that the birth of a healthy child will wipe out the trauma caused by the birth of an imperfect child. This is not so. Mothers do not forget such experiences. Emotional traumas that are not faced or resolved at the time they occur will continue to be destructive to the women who experience them, even when they have other, healthy children.

It is surely easier for family members and health professionals to encourage mothers who have had problem births to act as if nothing bad has happened and to focus their attention toward a new baby. But this does not help the mother recognize and cope with her intense disappointment by talking about it until she can learn to accept what has happened.

THE FATHER

Fathers may not feel as inadequate from a masculine point of view as their wives do as women when they do not produce healthy children. This difference is generally speculative, however, since in the past men have not shared their emotions about parenthood as openly as women. Now that our society is placing less emphasis on male-female differences, young men may feel encouraged to be more open about their reactions to parenthood. There already exists evidence that the same intensity of feeling occurs in both parents. It is interesting to note, for example, that the husbands of women who have abortions sometimes experience the same kind of depression that their wives feel.

There may be a marked difference between the way parents react to producing an abnormal baby. Fathers often feel alienated from the childbirth process, while at the same time they bear the traditional responsibility as the head of the family, caring for both the mother and the child. Many fathers suffer acutely from the idea that they bear the ultimate responsibility for what happens to their families.

At the same time health professionals tend to support this different sense of responsibility for fathers by their reliance on the mother as the parent primarily responsible for the child.

One mother, who was told in the delivery room that her baby was healthy, was visited three hours later—after her husband had left the hospital—and informed that the baby had Down syndrome. "Why didn't they call my husband?" the woman asked later. "Surely this news could have waited one hour until he was with me. But I guess physicians think only the mother is necessary."

The woman added, "I was terribly upset in that maternity ward. In the middle of everyone else's happiness, they just didn't know how to handle me. Clearly, it's not part of the training of medical people to help parents who've had a defective child."

Sensitive health care professionals will insist on dealing with both parents whenever possible in such situations. They will make an effort to be available for discussion at a time when the father can be present.

While mothers do biologically bear the child, there are, of course, certain inherited conditions in which the father's defective gene may be responsible for the child's abnormality. When transmission of the defective gene is clear-cut, the responsible parent understandably feels tremendous guilt. This is normal and to be expected. No amount of sympathy can alter the burden of this situation even when the biological facts indicate how the parent inherited the imperfect gene in the first place. But for a father who has not nurtured the child for nine months, yet still bears the responsibility for its imperfections, the sense of guilt for what he has done to the child and the mother can be overwhelming.

Fathers in this situation may need a great deal of help in order to be able to handle such burdens. As one father of a child with a genetic disease said, "The implication of genetic disease involves a powerful effect on the human psyche. It gets to the core of our being. It really hits us where it hurts, and we're not prepared for the attack."

HUSBAND AND WIFE

We have previously mentioned the contractual nature of marital relationships and the idea that any breakdown in the terms of the relationship may leave one or both partners feeling shortchanged. These tendencies extend not only to all aspects of the childbirth process but also to those situations in which a genetic defect is discovered in a family not specifically facing childbirth.

Defects in one's genetic makeup often account for negative feelings about oneself. Countless mothers who have faced problem births refer to what they felt as their resulting sense of "worthlessness." This diminished sense of oneself following the discovery of a genetic defect results in a state of mind that is extremely sensitive and easily hurt.

There is no way to predict how a couple will cope

when they have given birth to a child suffering the effects of a genetic disease. Some specialists believe that the most severe defects enable parents to deal more easily with the tragedy because they are not faced with caring for the child at home. Others believe the opposite is true.

Parents who have been unable to cope with such a tragedy tell us a lot about the emotional expense such an experience can have. One mother told of the "unnecessary wreckage" resulting from the birth of her child with Down syndrome. She referred to the fact that neither the professionals caring for her child, nor her husband, could face her sense of failure and loneliness brought on by the birth of the "bad baby." Despite the child's institutionalization and the birth of other, healthy children, the woman's marriage never recovered and in fact ended in divorce many years later.

When both partners are experiencing a similar sense of inadequacy, they are usually unable to be supportive of one another and they tend to be short-tempered, if not actually abusive. When a couple's deepest feelings and fears are withheld from each other there is little possibility of relief from such tension. Anger toward the other partner is the inevitable result.

One husband described the period following the birth of his Down syndrome daughter as a time when he felt he "was on a merry-go-round, going through the motions, but not feeling anything real."

The marital tensions resulting from the discovery of a genetic defect are often so severe that a high percentage of couples separate or divorce following such an experience. There is some evidence that the divorce rate among this group is four times higher than among the general public.

The distress parents experience when a defective child is born often prevents couples from maintaining their usual sexual relationship. This situation is sometimes further aggravated by the fear of another pregnancy. In such a marital relationship a vicious and destructive cycle may ensue: two sensitive, hurting individuals who now more than ever need the closeness of a strong relationship and an expression of physical love, find instead that their separate pain draws them apart to the point where they can no longer express that love. This sexual failure—in addition to the failure to produce a healthy child—tends to lower a couple's already weakened self-esteem. The mother of a child with a genetic defect wrote that her husband "had nightmares for some time after the baby's birth. He was not interested in having sexual relations for a long time."

Tammy and John's case is a good illustration of what often occurs in a couple's relationship after the birth of a genetically diseased baby. They first got help weeks after the birth of their Down syndrome baby, and for the first time the couple learned that John sincerely believed Tammy had been the cause of the problem because she carried "bad genes." Although John never actually said this to his wife, his coldness toward her had increased her own sense of inadequacy as a mother and as a woman.

What we have here is a perfect script for a soap opera: Tammy and John have a reasonably good marriage, but it is not perfect and each has his disappointments since the relationship is not as close as they expected. Their pregnancy was more or less planned to "bring them closer together" and to set their marriage on a steady course, free of the conflicts they had been experiencing with each other's large and intrusive families. Throughout her pregnancy Tammy began to feel fairly relaxed about herself as a person. She and John had fewer arguments and became more loving toward one another. For the first time in her life, Tammy even began to assert her independence from her mother, who was a very kind, but very demanding woman who wanted to be involved in every part of her daughter's life.

Then the earth fell in, as some have described the birth of a "bad" baby. John and Tammy are so disappointed in themselves, and in each other, that they are unable to talk to one another about this disturbing event. The couple is too frightened to consider the long-range problems of caring for the defective child. Tammy and John grow farther and farther apart. Each is depressed, but neither recognizes the signs of depression in the other, and each assumes that the depression is not shared by the mate. John has the escape of his job, which takes him away from home ten hours a day. But Tammy has no escape, and increasingly faces the anxiety of having neighbors see that her baby is "different." Thus, she feels she is publicly displaying the fact that she is, by her standards, an "inadequate woman."

Needless to say, if this scenario is carried to the seemingly inevitable conclusion, Tammy and John grow distant and they have no real emotional contact—not even the sexual relations that used to bring them together.

The script grinds on, with John finding himself another woman who makes him feel better about himself. She even helps bring back his dream of fathering normal children. Or, the script might show Tammy becoming so depressed that she can no longer care for the baby, and her mother assuming all responsibility for the child. This leaves her feeling even more inadequate. Eventually, of course, Tammy and John no longer have a relationship, and they separate.

What actually happened to Tammy and John is that they were referred for genetic counseling to determine their chances of having normal children in the future.

Through extensive discussions with John, the genetic counselor was able to learn about his distorted idea that Tammy had been the cause of his baby's abnormality. After genetic studies were done, the counselor explained to John that the defect was a genetic "accident," and was due to an extra chromosome the baby possessed.

The counselor also helped both John and Tammy recognize the depression they were experiencing and to see that this was a crucial and necessary phase for them to go through in order to be able to care for their baby, not to mention each other, responsibly. Since they had never heard of amniocentesis, or prenatal diagnosis, the counselor told them how any future pregnancies could be evaluated medically, and how they could be assured of not having another child with Down syndrome. Just learning that she still had the potential for producing a normal child did a lot to help Tammy over her depression.

After talking to both Tammy and John privately, the counselor spoke with the couple together and discussed their common emotional problems resulting from this family crisis. This counseling session began a pattern of communicating which was very important in John and Tammy's ability to work out the many problems they had to face in caring for their baby and in maintaining their marriage.

A MATTER OF GRIEF

When a person loses a loved one, and this would include the loss of an infant at birth or the birth of a child which is stillborn, the usual grief reaction lasts about six months, perhaps a little longer. But the parents of a handicapped child probably never stop mourning the lack of "normality" of their child. As a result, such parents may suffer a continuing grief, which becomes even more intense as their child fails to achieve certain normal milestones in the growth process.

The parents of a handicapped child may feel especially sad when their child fails to talk, walk, or ride a tricycle at the same time as a friend's youngster. Later in life, times for sadness may occur when the handicapped child does not begin school, or participate in little league sports, or begin dating when other youngsters his age do. At these times the parents of handicapped youngsters will need special support and understanding from each other, from friends, and from health care professionals.

Aside from this prolonged mourning which parents of handicapped youngsters often experience, these parents must also go through an immediate mourning process following the birth of the child and the identification of the handicap. In general, the stages in this process of mourning are shock, disbelief, and acceptance of grief.

An Albany Medical College team observes, however:

> Seldom do families progress smoothly from shock to disbelief to acceptance. Parents usually will experience varying periods of denial, during which they will refuse to accept either the diagnosis or their own feelings about the implications that a particular diagnosis has for their child. Such parents become very knowledgeable about their child's medical problem, yet they fail to come to grips with its emotional implications.

Sometimes parents will not be able to believe the medical facts that have been told to them about their child's case. It is not uncommon to find parents who are "shopping around" until they find someone who will tell them what they want to hear. As often as not, this individual will not be a bona fide health professional, but will be someone on the fringes of the health care community—someone who will want a great deal of money to administer some untested but highly touted dosage of vitamins, special foods, special chemicals, or even faith healing. Parents who have been deeply depressed by the birth of a handicapped child, and who are feeling a great deal of guilt, are vulnerable to the promises of these questionable practitioners, and should beware of them.

Another unhealthy reaction to mourning by the parents of a handicapped child is overprotection, or failure to encourage the child to develop as quickly as possible. According to an article in the *Journal of the American Academy of Family Physicians:*

> It is normal and appropriate for the parents of a handicapped child to have negative feelings. When parents do not understand this, they feel guilty and begin to overprotect their child. Overprotection tends to give the parents some measure of control over a difficult and frightening situation, but it also keeps the youngster at an infantile level and blocks his development in areas where he may not be handicapped.

CHILDREN

In families where there are children other than the one affected by a genetic defect, it is very important to be concerned with their reactions to what has just happened with the new baby.

Children of all ages need to be informed about what is happening in a family facing this kind of stress. Eventually these youngsters will learn the facts, and it is generally easier for everyone concerned if the truth is shared from the beginning. However, there are some situations in which the condition itself, or the age or emotional health of the siblings, do not warrant a complete disclosure. In these situations it is strongly recommended that the advice of the genetic counselor be sought, since the counselor's opinions are generally based on the experiences of numerous families with similar problems. In some situations it will be appropriate for the counselor to see the other children in the family for a regular counseling session in order to explain the disease.

Parents should be sensitive to the fact that just as they suffer from intense concern about their genetic makeup, so can their children. Teenage children, in particular, must be given every opportunity to reach a complete understanding of the situation and its relationship to their reproductive lives. This is often difficult and painful for parents; accordingly, they should be encouraged to seek additional counseling help, sometimes with their children along so that everyone in the family hears the same information. The long-term effect of this apprehension about their own reproductive capabilities can be devastating to children of all ages. Parents should always be sure that their children's anxieties over genetic risks are dealt with, whether or not they are openly expressed. Professional help from a therapist may be indicated for children facing this kind of severe family crisis. Consultations to determine the need for such help can be arranged through the family physician, the genetic counselor, or the family service agency in most communities.

One young girl told her counselor, "My feelings about my [retarded] sister are so complicated. I feel so lucky that it wasn't me. And that makes me feel pretty guilty."

Many parents and youngsters feel a strong sense of shame when a genetic disease is diagnosed in themselves, their children, or their siblings. Many parents of affected children are unable to tell their friends what has happened. Staying away from these friends makes it easier to maintain this denial. Teenage siblings of affected children may be embarrassed to have their friends know about or see the affected child, and may draw away from friends to avoid such exposure. These children sometimes feel very "different" from their friends.

One man revealed that as he was growing up his brother's genetic illness made him feel that he, too, was defective, but that it "just didn't show."

Some of the feelings coming into play among the brothers and sisters of children who have been diagnosed as suffering from a genetically determined disease may be:

—Did my angry wishes in response to my parents having more children cause this illness?
—Do I have the same problem?
—Will my children have the same problem?
—What will my friends say when they see my baby brother or sister is so queer?
—Is this condition catching?
—Will I have to take care of this brother or sister when my parents die?
—Does our family have bad blood?

Older children should be told when they may be carriers of a genetic disease. Some adults will argue that the anxiety produced by this knowledge of genetic risk will be more harmful than the failure to know the risks.

We do not believe in this reasoning, and would encourage parents to help their children learn to deal with their particular genetic problem, to see that they understand the genetic pattern responsible for the problem, and that they have the opportunity to talk about it freely in the protective atmosphere of their family.

The Whartons were faced with such a problem when their sixteen-year-old son Ralph, who has suffered from cystic fibrosis for most of his life, began to show great interest in girls and to date regularly. Ralph's disease was quite manageable, but nevertheless his chances of fathering children were limited. The Whartons realized this could be a matter of great concern to their son and knew they would have to discuss it with him. But when? Wouldn't the discussion be dangerous, even destructive, especially at this time when he was first expressing serious interest in young women? Should the Whartons wait until Ralph was ready to go off to college?

Ralph's parents knew that the task ahead of them would never have a perfect time, nor would it be easy. They decided to speak to their doctor, who knew Ralph well and who might have had experience with other cystic fibrosis youngsters Ralph's age.

The doctor agreed that Ralph should be told of the problem. He offered to see Ralph himself to answer any questions his parents couldn't handle.

Although the experience was painful for everyone involved, Ralph learned to talk about the angry feelings that were aroused in him, and eventually the whole family was able to make peace with their bad luck. Today Ralph is the proud father of two adopted children.

To illustrate what can happen if this kind of information is not shared, Dr. Aubrey Milunsky of the Massachusetts General Hospital has cited three different families in which the wife had discovered only after becoming pregnant that she had a sibling with Down syndrome. If the parents of these women had informed them beforehand, each would have been able to seek genetic counseling in order to learn about the chances of giving birth to a child with this disorder, and how to avoid it.

Parents who find themselves discussing such sensitive matters with their children should be prepared to be faced with possible anger from the children, who may perceive the defect as a "burden" foisted upon them by the parents. In time, however, sympathetic parents who are able to communicate with their children, particularly as they mature, should be able to discuss the alternative approaches to parenthood which their children can consider despite the genetic problems they face.

Some of these alternatives may be: prenatal diagnosis coupled with abortion if necessary; adoption; and carrier testing (genetic screening) of marital partners. Another viable alternative may be artificial insemination, which involves the use of sperm from an anonymous male donor who has no detectable genetic illnesses, to fertilize a woman whose husband does have a genetic illness that might be transmitted to offspring. This procedure allows couples to have the partial experience of bearing their own children and has been used with considerable success by many couples.

All of these alternative possibilities carry heavy emotional burdens which must be considered in making the eventual decision to select one alternative rather than another.

GRANDPARENTS

Grandparents of a baby born with a defect often suffer intensely, too, perhaps because of the biological involvement they sense, but may not fully understand. In some cases, when grandparents realize an infant suffers from a familial disease, there is a special kind of guilt that can result from many years of "keeping the family secret." Even in the case of a new mutation or accident resulting in a defective child, grandparents sometimes experience strong feelings that they are responsible. Or each side of the family may be totally convinced that the other side is responsible for the defect.

One mother says that her parents "were never the same" after her daughter was born with a fatal defect. She felt that she saw her mother "age before my very eyes," when she was told that the baby could not live.

Sometimes grandparents are perfectionists, and the tangible proof that their children have been imperfect enough to produce a defective grandchild is a real blow to their own ego. Another mother of a defective child spoke of her parents' horror at what happened to her and commented that perhaps there was something to the biblical statement that "the sins of the fathers are visited on the child."

In closely knit families, it is important to explain the genetics that caused the birth of an affected child to all members, grandparents included. Although this may be difficult to arrange, it is important because of the need to obtain accurate family histories.

The natural tendency to denial that grandparents may persist in is usually irritating to other family members, and especially to the distraught parents who really need help in learning to live with the reality of their affected child. Grandparents who refuse to accept the diagnosis often cling to straws. They may make statements such as, "I'm sure she'll grow out of it," or "She looks so normal, I'm sure they made a mistake at that hospital."

When the parents have siblings, informed grandparents can take responsibility for notifying them that they may also be at risk for the same condition. Parents who learn unexpectedly that their family carries the gene for a heritable defect will probably want to share this information with brothers or sisters who are also at risk. This is not always easy to do, because of the strong feelings people have about their genes. To be rejected by a sibling for trying to act responsibly toward him or her can be particularly upsetting when one already is suffering from the burden of discovery about oneself or one's offspring.

8

**A LOOK
AT SOME
GENETIC
DISEASES**

IN AN EARLIER CHAPTER WE TALKED ABOUT THE BASIC kinds of genetic disorders: the chromosome disorders, the disorders caused by single pairs of genes, and the disorders caused by a number of pairs of genes and their interactions with the environment.

Since there are enough different genetic diseases to fill several volumes with descriptions and case histories, we do not intend to dwell on such specifics.

At this point, therefore, we are going to discuss only a few of the most talked-about—but perhaps least understood—genetic diseases. There are extensive reference materials available for any particular genetic disease, and such information can be obtained from many of the sources listed in the appendix of this book, or from the vertical file of your local library.

THE GENETIC CONNECTION

DOWN SYNDROME

Betty and Andrew Farina had been married for eighteen years. They were the parents of a normal, healthy twelve-year-old son. At age thirty-nine Betty became pregnant again.

When she was about two months pregnant Betty visited her obstetrician, the same doctor who had delivered her first child. The obstetrician expressed concern over the pregnancy because of Mrs. Farina's age. He discussed some possible problems with her, and suggested that the pregnancy be terminated.

Mrs. Farina already had heard of the prenatal test called amniocentesis, and to learn more about it she sought the advice of two other obstetricians. At the time, however, most obstetricians were wary of performing amniocentesis, since they were uncertain about potential complications of the procedure in which a small amount of amniotic fluid is withdrawn from the cavity around the fetus. Within this fluid float cells which originated with the fetus and can therefore be tested to determine the chromosome makeup of the developing person. Today, physicians have learned that amniocentesis is not only an effective method of testing for a number of genetic diseases, but it is also a safe procedure.

But without the information amniocentesis could provide, Mrs. Farina decided to go ahead with the pregnancy in spite of the fact that she had been worried about its outcome ever since her very first visit to the doctor.

Mrs. Farina gave birth to Barry on January 17, 1974, after a short, eight-month pregnancy. The child's birth weight was 5 pounds, 11 ounces. One can imagine the Farinas' relief when, immediately after the birth, they were told that the child was "fine."

Four hours later, however, the pediatrician spoke to Andrew Farina and told him, "I have some bad news for you. Your baby has Down syndrome."

Mr. Farina did not know what that meant, and he asked the doctor: "Is the baby all right?" The reply was "yes," meaning that the child's general physical health was good in spite of the inborn disease.

Mr. Farina soon reported the doctor's statement to his wife, who immediately realized the child was "mongoloid," and she became distraught. Andrew was dumbfounded, since only four hours earlier he had been told that his wife had delivered a normal son.

The experience that Mr. and Mrs. Farina went through, while unfortunate, is not all that unusual when a child with Down syndrome is born. Unlike many of the genetic diseases—such as thalassemia, sickle-cell disease, Tay Sachs disease and others—Down syndrome can usually be identified relatively quickly, at least during the first few weeks of life, if not in the first few hours.

As Australian pediatrician Dr. David Pitt has noted: "At first the baby [with Down syndrome] may look like any average baby, and the special features may not be noticed until seen by an alert nurse or doctor."

The fact is, however, as Dr. Pitt points out,

A Down syndrome baby is "born different." . . . He is different both physically and mentally from a normal baby. The physical differences consist of some reduction in body and head size, and some physical characteristics which can usually be recognized at birth. The eyes are a little different, particularly in their upward and outward slope, the ears may be small, the tongue may be big, the hands and feet may have distinctive shapes. These characteristics, especially the small head, often become more obvious as the child grows older.

This "syndrome" was first described as a distinct disease in 1866 by British physician Dr. Langdon Down, hence the name the syndrome now carries. Dr. Down also observed that victims of this disease, with their slanting eyes, seemed to resemble Orientals, thus they were referred to as "mongoloids," "mongols," and even "mongolian idiots." These adjectives were never intended as racial or ethnic slurs on Orientals, but merely were used as a convenient description. However, the designation has been interpreted as racist, not to mention its unpleasant connotation for the parents of affected youngsters. For these reasons, it is vastly preferred that the name Down syndrome, and never "mongoloid," be used to refer to affected individuals.

The chances of bearing a child with Down syndrome rise significantly with the mother's age. It is well-documented, however, that there is a sharp increase in the incidence of the disease in mothers older than thirty-five, and an even sharper increase after age forty. In fact, the chances of bearing a baby with Down syndrome when a woman is between thirty and thirty-four years old are about 1 in 750; between ages thirty-five and thirty-nine the chance is about 1 in 300; between forty and forty-four the chance is about 1 in 80; and after a woman is forty-five years old the chance of her bearing an affected child jumps to about 1 in 40. On the other hand, women under thirty years of age have only about 1 chance in 1,500 of having a child with Down syndrome.

The precise reason for the drastic increase in incidence of Down syndrome babies born to older women is not yet known for certain. And questions have been asked about whether this same phenomenon holds true for older fathers who sire children. There have been mixed data on this matter, but recent studies have shown an apparent jump in risk for offspring of fathers who are fifty-five years of age or older. In any case, the mechanisms of this possible effect of older fathers, or even of the well-documented effect of older mothers, are not clearly understood.

One theory is attributed to the significant difference in the way eggs and sperm are produced. From the time of her birth, as we mentioned earlier, the mother's body has contained a lifetime supply of eggs—several hundred thousand. These eggs reside in the periphery of the ovaries, and await their turns for ovulation. Every month after menstruation begins, about one hundred eggs begin to mature, but only one egg actually bursts free and becomes available for fertilization, leaving the remainder to degenerate.

Consequently, the supply of eggs diminishes each month. Over the years, those eggs which remain in the ovaries are subjected to a number of environmental influences such as X rays, ionospheric irradiation, and various other pollutants—as well as simply age—and all of these factors may damage the genetic material in the eggs. Obviously, then, the eggs which have lingered in a woman's body for forty or fifty years may be more vulnerable than those which have existed only for half that time.

Male sperm, on the other hand, are not manufactured until the time of puberty. The supply of sperm is being renewed constantly, regardless of a man's age. It is possible, however, that as a man's sexual organs begin to age, there is a higher chance of error in manufacturing new sperm cells. Only future research will help to define more fully the relationship between paternal age and chromosomal defects.

At any rate, we now know that the vast majority (95 to 98 percent) of cases of Down syndrome are associated with an extra chromosome. Instead of the usual complement of 46 chromosomes, the victim of Down syndrome carries 47 chromosomes in each body cell.

Ordinarily, as we discussed back in Chapter 2, a sperm cell with 23 chromosomes fertilizes an egg with 23 chromosomes, thus forming a new cell with 46 chromosomes. This cell duplicates itself billions of times until a new human being is formed—with each of that new individual's cells carrying exact replicas of those original 46 chromosomes.

If, however, a sperm or an egg has received some extra genetic material when it was originally produced, it may have 24 chromosomes instead of the normal 23. Thus, when a sperm with 23 chromosomes combines with an egg that has 24, the result is a new cell of 47 chromosomes. Since each of the body cells of the person-to-be will contain exact carbon copies of this original genetic material, they all will contain 47 chromosomes. Somehow the presence of this extra genetic material disturbs the usual orderly development of the body and the brain.

When physicians sort and count the chromosomes of a victim of Down syndrome, they often find the usual pair of chromosomes in 22 of the 23 normal pairs. One chromosome pair, however, occurs as a trio instead—chromosome number 21—and this accounts for the damaging forty-seventh chromosome. Thus this form of Down syndrome is referred to as trisomy 21.

Another type of genetic abnormality occurs in about 4 percent of Down syndrome victims. This is called "translocation." In this form of the disease, victims also have an extra chromosome number 21. But instead of being found with the other chromosomes of this number, this extra chromosome has broken off and attached itself to another chromosome.

This type of Down syndrome is usually inherited from the parents rather than being a genetic "accident" near the time of conception. Parents can carry a translocated chromosome number 21 within their own cells without showing any symptoms of Down syndrome. This is possible since the affected parent still carries the correct amount of genetic material, even though some of it is translocated—or in the wrong place. Thus when that parent's body cells divide to produce the sex cells (sperm or eggs), they may contain the normal chromosome number 21 as well as the translocated chromosome number 21, thereby giving the offspring too much chromosome-21 material. The outward results are virtually the same as those seen in victims of the trisomy-21 form of Down syndrome. Down syndrome caused by "translocation" can be detected in the parents by a chromosome test.

The third genetic type of Down syndrome is very rare and is called "mosaicism." It occurs when some of the victim's cells have 46 chromosomes and others have 47 chromosomes. This type of the disease is usually not carried by the parents, but probably results from an accident early in the cell division of the fertilized egg. Babies with this form of Down syndrome may have only some of the features of the syndrome, since only some of their cells have an abnormal number of chromosomes.

One of the most serious problems faced by children with Down syndrome—and their parents—is mental retardation.

Babies with Down syndrome are often slow in developing even the most basic motor skills, such as learning to turn over, sit up, crawl, walk, and speak. Even when their early development is fairly normal, the retardation will be noticed eventually. Children with Down syndrome may never reach anything near normal intelligence. In fact, most children with Down syndrome have IQs in the thirties to fifties, though occasionally the range reaches into the sixties and seventies. (Average IQ scores for normal children are in the range of 90 to 110.)

Furthermore, these children with Down syndrome seem to have a greater number of heart defects, and are far more susceptible to colds and respiratory infections than normal infants, and their chances of getting leukemia are about three times those of normal children.

When a child with Down syndrome survives the first few years of life, the death rates become approximately the same as for normal persons until about age forty. Since victims of Down syndrome seem to age more rapidly than normal children do, by the time they reach the age of forty or thereabouts they sometimes become susceptible to diseases usually associated with "old age."

There is no known "cure" for Down syndrome at present. It is possible, however, to drastically curtail the chances of bearing such affected children through a proper course of counseling and prenatal diagnosis. Amniocentesis, for example, can help the physician spot a fetus with Down syndrome, and the pregnancy can be terminated. Since conceiving one child with Down syndrome does not mean other children will necessarily be so affected, the couple can, after counseling, choose to try again. Indeed, the recurrence risk for the most common type of Down syndrome is only 1 percent for women up to age thirty-five.

Not every pregnant woman needs to undergo these tests, since there are a number of factors that can help pinpoint couples who may be at risk for bearing a child with Down syndrome. You are at risk and should have amniocentesis if:

—A pregnant wife is older than age thirty-five. (If the husband is fifty-five years of age or older, consult a genetics center and ask about current recommended procedure.)

—You are already parents of one child with Down syndrome or some other chromosome abnormality.

((167))

THE GENETIC CONNECTION

—Your family is known to have a specific genetic defect that can be detected by prenatal diagnosis.

—You are a woman known to be a carrier of a disorder that affects males only.

—Either parent is a known carrier for a chromosome abnormality.

HUNTINGTON'S DISEASE

Perhaps the greatest tragedy of Huntington's disease is that a person usually doesn't know that he or she is a victim of this devastating central nervous system disorder until adulthood. Often this means that such persons already have had children of their own—and may unknowingly have passed it along to these offspring.

In the past—and even today—when the diagnosis of Huntington's disease has not yet been determined in an individual, it is often confused with alcoholism or a "mental" disorder. Generations ago, victims of Huntington's disease were thought to be possessed by devils and were sometimes burned at the stake. Such "shame," occasionally still referred to as a "family curse," or "that disease," has often caused families to successfully hide the existence of the disease in their families for hundreds of years. Because of this shame and guilt, the actual prevalence of Huntington's disease is somewhat vague. (The same phenomenon occurs with many other genetic diseases, and has been one of the reasons they are often difficult for scientists to trace.)

Because of the lack of knowledge even among the victims of the disease, many children of parents who have Huntington's disease never had the benefit of knowing that they, too, were at risk for developing it. And they are also at risk for passing it along to 50 percent of their own children.

Legendary American folk singer Woody Guthrie is perhaps the most famous victim of Huntington's disease. In his early forties Woody began to develop the symptoms of Huntington's disease. He died fifteen years later, in 1967, after having spent a number of years bedridden and immobile, unable even to communicate except by blinking his eyes. And like many other victims of Huntington's disease, Woody already had fathered three children—Arlo, Joady, and Nora—before he knew about the deadly legacy he might be leaving them.

If some good can possibly come out of this kind of tragedy, then in the Guthries' case it has indeed. Woody's second wife, Marjorie, has devoted both her life and her family's resources to educating the public— as well as the professionals—about Huntington's disease.

Woody once said, "I hate a song that makes you think that you're just born to lose . . ."

Says Marjorie Guthrie today, "I am out to fight those kinds of songs to my very last breath, and my last drop of blood." As the guiding force behind the Committee to Combat Huntington's Disease, based in New York City, Marjorie is doing just that. She spends her time counseling families who have just learned they are at risk—or victims—of Huntington's disease, she testifies before Congress on behalf of funding to study the causes of genetic diseases and to provide counseling for families they affect, and she travels all over the world setting up local chapters of her CCHD.

Huntington's disease used to be called Huntington's

chorea. It was originally referred to as hereditary chorea
by an American doctor, George Huntington, who wrote
an essay "On Chorea" in an 1872 edition of *The Medical and Surgical Reporter*. The name "chorea" comes
from the Greek word for dance. The dance, in Dr.
Huntington's words, refers to

> the irregular and spasmodic action of certain muscles, as
> of the face, arms, etc. These movements gradually increase, when muscles hitherto unaffected take on the
> spasmodic action, until every muscle in the body becomes
> affected . . . and the poor patient presents a spectacle
> which is anything but pleasing to witness.

Dr. Huntington's observations of this disease more
than a hundred years ago were so keen that they can
be repeated today with few, if any, corrections.

> The hereditary chorea, as I shall call it, is confined to
> certain and fortunately a few families, and has been
> transmitted to them, an heirloom from generations away
> back in the dim past. It is spoken of by those in whose
> veins the seeds of the disease are known to exist, with a
> kind of horror and not at all alluded to except through
> dire necessity, when it is mentioned as "that disorder."
> [It] hardly ever [manifests] itself until adult or middle
> life, and then [comes] on gradually but surely, increasing
> by degrees, and often occupying years in its development,
> until the hapless sufferer is but a quivering wreck of his
> former self.
> Unstable and whimsical as the disease may be in *other*
> respects, in this it is firm, it never skips a generation to
> again manifest itself in another; once having yielded its
> claims, it never regains them.

Thus even before Mendel's laws of heredity became

generally accepted in 1900, Dr. Huntington had described perfectly the mode of transmission of this disease, a dominant disorder|(see pages 42–43). This means that there are no "carriers" of the disease, such as the carriers of Tay Sachs disease or hemophilia, who do not suffer it themselves. Every person that carries the gene for Huntington's disease will, if he or she lives long enough, suffer the disease itself. And every offspring of such a person—both male and female—has a 50-percent chance of developing the disease later in life.

When Dr. Huntington first described this hereditary chorea, he was mainly aware of the physical contortions and uncontrollable movements with which its victims were stricken. Since that time, however, it has been observed that some victims of the disease do not initially suffer from the chorea. Instead Huntington's disease may begin with personality changes such as irritability, indifference, poor judgment, forgetfulness, and carelessness about personal appearance and commitments.

The progressive deterioration of the central nervous system leads to rapid decline in the ability to control body movements, and the mental deterioration can become severe. Victims often live from five to fifteen years with Huntington's disease after it develops, many of those years being spent helplessly in bed.

Frequently, Huntington's disease victims are first diagnosed as having a mental disorder. Indeed, many Huntington's disease victims are hospitalized for "mental illness" before the correct diagnosis is made.

This is exactly what happened to a young man we'll call Mark. He was quite unusual in that he developed

Huntington's disease while he was still a teenager. In all other ways, however, Huntington's disease victims often go through the same medical maze that Mark and his family did.

His stepfather tells the story:

> At 14 he ran away for the first time. He went to his grandfather's farm. I tried to reason with him at this point and he did seem to respond. But about a month later he stole a pickup and ran away. He had a pretty bad wreck and it cost us about a thousand dollars in damage. We had him admitted to [a nearby] hospital for observation and treatment of a possible mental disorder. He was soon transferred to a larger, long-term psychiatric hospital, where he remained for a year.
>
> He enlisted in the Marines when he was seventeen. But he got in trouble and received a bad conduct discharge.
>
> It wasn't until three years later that we found out for the first time that he might be suffering from Huntington's disease. Since then we have found out just how fortunate we are. First of all, the Huntington's disease came from his real father's side of the family. We could never contact him, but we found out that his real father's father died from Huntington's disease in the very hospital our son had stayed in for ten months!
>
> It really amazes me to think that poor Mark could have been treated at the very best hospital this nation has to offer for a total of almost five years and during this time not one doctor even hinted to me or my wife that something physical was wrong with our son.

In spite of the physical and mental changes wrought by Huntington's disease, and the inability of victims to communicate, it is possible that the victim's actual mental capacity may remain unaffected—a normal mind held captive in a body that simply won't respond to its orders. Marjorie Guthrie recalls, "Woody's mind was sharp until the end. That's one of the many misconceptions about Huntington's disease—that the victim's mental powers always fail. Often, they remain intact."

You are at risk for having a child with Huntington's disease if either of your parents or your spouse's parents have suffered the disease, or if either of you, the prospective parents, have it.

Families who suspect that they are at risk for Huntington's disease will vary in their ability to deal with the burden of this uncertainty. Adolescents with an affected parent should be given adequate genetic counseling so they will understand the nature of their risk. In addition to the need to deal with the facts, adolescents as well as adults at risk for Huntington's disease need considerable emotional support to adjust to such a burden and to achieve as normal a life as possible.

At the present time there is no known cure for this disease, nor is there a method to predict its presence in an individual. Genetic counseling for families with Huntington's disease can only explain the disease and the risks of developing it, as well as allowing individuals to discuss the conflicts they feel.

CYSTIC FIBROSIS

"Outwardly, Chris doesn't appear to be suffering from a serious disorder. The only indications that she is ill may be her thin, small build, slightly protruding abdomen, discolored teeth and enlarged fingertips—all not very conspicuous. But appearances are often deceptive . . ."

The very fact that appearances *are* often deceptive, coupled with a general misunderstanding of the disease and its consequences, simply help make cystic fibrosis all the more dangerous.

Cystic fibrosis is not merely misunderstood. Few persons seem to know much about it at all. An informal survey among well-educated professionals was informative in this respect.

One young man asked if cystic fibrosis wasn't "a kind of paralysis, something like polio."

A woman with a master's degree in business asked, "Isn't that when you get lumps all over your body?"

And when a secretary in a large New York office was asked, "Did you ever hear of cystic fibrosis," she stepped back two steps, quickly covered her mouth and nose with her hand, and replied: "Yes, it's catching, isn't it?"

No.

None of the above is remotely near being a correct description of cystic fibrosis—the most common fatal genetic disease of children. One reason for the confusion may be that cystic fibrosis itself is a great masquerader. Its symptoms have frequently been mistaken for other diseases—the cough of cystic fibrosis may sound like whooping cough, and the wheezing may be mistaken for asthma. Several digestive problems also mimic the intestinal symptoms of cystic fibrosis.

The disease itself affects the functioning of certain glands—called the exocrine glands. These are the glands that secrete mucus and sweat, tears and saliva. The mucus that is secreted by the body of a cystic fibrosis victim is abnormally thick and gluey. Instead of the usual thin, runny mucus, which helps keep the lungs and the breathing tubes free of dust and dirt, the mucus of the cystic fibrosis victim actually makes it harder to breathe. This thick mucus often clogs the breathing passages, and traps air as well as germs, which can become infected and cause serious problems. Sweat glands in the cystic fibrosis victim also go awry, secreting sweat that is extremely salty.

Cystic fibrosis wasn't identified until 1938, and at the time it was invariably considered fatal within a relatively brief period. Indeed, the correct diagnosis was often not made until the victim already had died and an autopsy was performed.

Even as recently as 1973, the prestigious British medical journal, *The Lancet,* carried an article on the disease which pointed out that "Awareness of the disease seems to have spread rather slowly, and probably some patients are still being misdiagnosed . . ."

Notes the same article: "Although life expectancy for those with the condition seems to be improving, it is still an important cause of childhood morbidity and mortality, some of which may be preventable."

It wasn't such a long time ago that cystic fibrosis was considered quite rare. Today, however, it is estimated that a new case of the disease occurs in about 1 in every 1,600 live births. Although treatment for cystic fibrosis is becoming more effective—there is no known cure—it remains a significant cause of childhood deaths. Cystic fibrosis kills more children than any other genetic disease.

It is estimated today that about one in every twenty persons carries at least one gene for cystic fibrosis. This is equal to about ten million people in the United

States. Cystic fibrosis mainly affects white people. The "carriers" of at least one gene for cystic fibrosis are so common that marriages between them often occur—statistically about once in every 400 marriages.

Since cystic fibrosis is a hereditary disease transmitted through *recessive* inheritance (see chapter 2), a person must possess two separate cystic fibrosis genes before becoming a victim of the disease. Cystic fibrosis is equally likely to affect males and females, and it is not affected by order of birth. A person can be born with the disease only when both parents are carriers (or victims) of cystic fibrosis.

As with most recessive genetic diseases, those who merely carry a single gene are not affected by symptoms. Unlike some diseases, however, there is no test to detect the carriers of the cystic fibrosis gene at this time. Thus, an individual's status as a carrier cannot be recognized and confirmed until that person becomes a parent of a child with the disease. Of course any family history of cystic fibrosis can tip off health professionals to be aware of the possibility that an individual may be a carrier.

The actual cause of cystic fibrosis is not known even today. Common symptoms of the disease include the specific problems with the lungs, as well as difficulties with digestion. Different victims are affected by cystic fibrosis in different ways, and with varying degrees of severity.

In some victims cystic fibrosis affects primarily the lungs, with the sticky mucus making it difficult to breathe. Other cystic fibrosis victims suffer when the thick mucus blocks the flow of natural secretions from the pancreas gland and causes small lumps, or cysts, to form. These cysts often cause obstruction and scarring (or fibrosis) of the pancreas. Hence the disease received its original name, "cystic fibrosis of the pancreas."

Today doctors know that the pancreas is not the only part of the body which is affected by this disease. Nevertheless, the early name it received continues to be used. Some doctors in other countries refer to cystic fibrosis as mucoviscidosis, because of the very thick (or viscid) mucus.

Often the symptoms of cystic fibrosis are not very obvious in young children. The particular combination of signs indicating the presence of cystic fibrosis include frequent cough, recurrent pneumonia, unusually large appetite, frequent bowel movements, small stature and enlarged fingertips.

The cough associated with cystic fibrosis can be particularly troublesome in a child's relationships at school and with friends. Mrs. H., mother of Tommy, a four-year-old cystic fibrosis victim, complains that she constantly has to tell the parents of Tommy's friends that his cough is not the symptom of a contagious illness. "I get very upset because Tommy is not invited to parties or outings with the other children because of this, and also because my son can't eat most of the food other kids eat because of his intestinal problems. It's so difficult to try to provide a child with some kind of a normal life when we are met with so much resistance by outsiders."

(It is not desirable to try to prevent or restrain the cystic fibrosis victim from coughing, since it is this natural reflex that helps remove the dangerous thick mucus from the lungs.)

Doctors diagnose cystic fibrosis with a couple of specific tests. One of them measures the amount of salt in the perspiration. Cystic fibrosis victims have very salty perspiration—indeed, mothers or grandmothers have often tipped off the doctors about a child's cystic fibrosis when they report that the infant tastes very salty when kissed. Another test analyzes the enzymes present in the intestinal tract to determine whether the pancreas is functioning properly.

Not so many years ago, cystic fibrosis was invariably fatal at an early age. Today, however, a good deal of progress has been made in treating victims of the disease. Perhaps most important in helping the cystic fibrosis victim to live a long and nearly normal life is early diagnosis, which allows for quick and modern management of the disease.

There is no specific course of treatment for cystic fibrosis, because there is a good deal of variation in the severity and course of the disease.

Among the treatments used are antibiotics, which fight or prevent lung infections, and various medications—taken by mouth or aerosol—which are used to thin and loosen the thick mucus, and to prevent it from clogging the tiny tubes of the lungs. Another effective method of clearing the lungs is known as "postural drainage," in which the child is put in certain positions to help drain various areas of the lungs. The parent or therapist may also gently clap or vibrate the chest wall to dislodge the small mucus plugs which form in the airways.

Because of these and other effective methods of treatment, many victims of cystic fibrosis can lead nearly normal lives. Among them are individuals such as Peter, who, according to the Cystic Fibrosis Foundation, is in his late twenties and "was an honor student in high school despite poor attendance because of illness. He went on to college to earn a degree in accounting. Today he holds a full-time job as a bookkeeper and is an ardent camper and skier."

Another cystic fibrosis victim is thirty-eight-year-old Harold. He is "a high school teacher, married, with one adopted child. A law school graduate, he decided after a number of years in practice to switch to the field he preferred."

The very medical progress that has allowed cystic fibrosis patients such as Peter and Harold to live to adulthood has, in another way, provided some more complications. In the days when cystic fibrosis victims invariably died young, there was no significant worry about the disease being passed along by victims—only when two carriers married could such a problem arise.

Now that an increasing number of persons with cystic fibrosis are living well into their reproductive years they must carefully consider all the factors before deciding to have children. If an individual with cystic fibrosis marries a cystic fibrosis carrier, 50 percent of the offspring can be expected to have the disease, and *all* non-victims will be carriers. But if two carriers marry, only 25 percent of the offspring can be expected to have cystic fibrosis, 50 percent of the children will be carriers, and 25 percent of the children will be normal.

Thus, when a cystic fibrosis victim becomes a parent

—a rare, but not impossible event—there is a significantly higher chance that the children will suffer the serious effects of this disease.

Here is a list of risks for bearing a child with cystic fibrosis, provided by the Cystic Fibrosis Foundation.

PARENTS	RISK FOR EACH PREGNANCY
Both parents known carriers	1 in 4
One parent is a sibling of an individual with CF; the other parent is a known carrier	1 in 6
Both parents are siblings of individuals with CF	1 in 9
One parent is an individual with CF; other parent has no known family history of CF	1 in 40
One parent is a known carrier of CF gene; other parent has no known family history of CF	1 in 80
One parent is a sibling of an individual with CF; other parent has no known family history of CF	1 in 120
One parent is an aunt or uncle of an individual with CF; other parent has no known family history of CF	1 in 120 to 1 in 160
Both parents are members of the general population—they have no known family history of CF	1 in 1,600

(This listing shows the variable risks that a child will inherit cystic fibrosis itself. The odds that a child may become a carrier of the cystic fibrosis gene are different.)

TAY SACHS DISEASE

Tay Sachs disease is known as the "Jewish disease," although even most Jewish persons had never heard of it until just a few years ago.

Nobody knows why this genetic disease, which invariably kills its victims before they reach their fourth or fifth birthdays, mainly strikes Jews of Eastern European origin. Only about 15 percent of the cases of Tay Sachs disease occur in other ethnic groups.

When they are born, these children appear to be normal. But because of an enzyme deficiency which causes brain deterioration, normal development stops at about six months of age. It is at this time that the victim of Tay Sachs disease begins to waste away. Slowly the infant begins to lose the newfound skills and coordination it has only just begun to acquire. Tragically, there is simply no hope. Nothing at all can be done for these youngsters, beyond keeping them as comfortable as possible until the end. Science has yet to discover either cure or treatment for Tay Sachs disease.

While there is as yet no known cure or treatment, Tay Sachs disease *can* be prevented. It is one of the genetic diseases for which safe and effective screening tests have been devised. Tay Sachs disease can not only be screened for, it can also be detected *in utero;* that is, if a woman is pregnant, the fetus can be tested for the disease via amniocentesis. If the test is positive, the parents may choose to have the fetus aborted so neither child nor family will have to face the traumatic suffering.

About 1 in every 25 Jews of Eastern European origin carries the faulty gene responsible for Tay Sachs disease. The odds among the non-Jewish population or among Jews who aren't from Eastern Europe for being a carrier are 1 in 300. (However, because of intermarriages between Jewish people from around the world it is suggested that all Jews be screened for Tay Sachs disease.) Since Tay Sachs is another disease governed by recessive inheritance characteristics (see Chapter 2), these carrier parents do not have the disease; they only carry the potential to pass it along to their offspring. Indeed, once in about every 625 marriages, two carriers of the faulty gene are brought together.

The faulty gene that causes development of Tay Sachs disease is defective because it fails to tell the body to produce an enzyme called hexosaminidase A, or Hex-A for short. This enzyme helps break down fatty materials (called sphingolipids) that accumulate within the cells of the brain and nervous system. When the fats accumulate for too long, they begin to choke and destroy the cells. The result is loss of coordination, seizures, blindness, and eventual death.

Incidentally, there are a number of other recessive genetic diseases which are quite similar to Tay Sachs disease, and affect the same ethnic populations. These diseases are known as sphingolipidoses, and include diseases with names like Gaucher's disease and Niemann-

Pick disease. They are caused by lack of other enzymes. Unfortunately there is not yet a method of detecting carriers of these diseases, as can be done in Tay Sachs disease. These diseases are, however, susceptible to prenatal diagnosis by amniocentesis.

Even though there is no cure for Tay Sachs disease, scientists hope that someday it can be eliminated by advance identification and counseling of carriers. Unfortunately, records show that 82 percent of babies born with Tay Sachs disease are born into families which have no prior history of the illness. Thus, unlike many other genetic diseases, there is often no alerting signal to possible carriers of this disease.

For this reason, physicians recommend that all Jews of East European or Ashkenazic ancestry undergo the screening blood test for Tay Sachs disease. These tests are available in most communities, and are simply a matter of having a small amount of blood taken from one's arm and analyzed at a laboratory. Carriers of the gene for Tay Sachs disease are identified with a high degree of accuracy.

If a couple has learned that both members are carriers of the Tay Sachs gene, they usually decide that the woman will undergo amniocentesis with each pregnancy since they have a 50-percent risk of having a child with this fatal disease. If the test is positive, the parents can consider a termination of the pregnancy. Even though Tay Sachs disease is relatively rare, most parents would prefer to eliminate even the remote possibility by learning, first, if they carry the gene and then having the prenatal test when they become pregnant.

THE GENETIC CONNECTION

You may be at risk for Tay Sachs disease if you are a Jewish person descended from East European (Ashkenazic) ancestors. To eliminate the risk of bearing a child with Tay Sachs disease you must:

1 / Undergo the simple blood test to detect carriers.

2 / Obtain genetic counseling if the test is positive.

SICKLE-CELL ANEMIA

It's a real irony of evolution that the changes in the red blood cells that cause sickle-cell anemia apparently evolved thousands of years ago as a protective mechanism against another severe disease, malaria.

According to Yale University hematologist Dr. Howard A. Pearson, "The sickle gene is believed to have arisen by spontaneous mutation thousands of years ago in equatorial Africa. It has been convincingly demonstrated that the person with sickle-cell trait has an enhanced resistance to infection by the malaria parasite."

Thus, the mutation that caused the sickled red blood cells which result in so much trouble today was possibly a lifesaving change millennia ago. Individuals who possessed the sickled cells were better able to survive in the malaria-infested areas, and thus evolution favored them and their offspring. In strong support of this theory is the fact that in some parts of Western Africa, where malaria is endemic, the sickle-cell trait is still found in 40 percent of the population. In the United States, however, and in other countries where malaria has been wiped out and the sickle-cell trait is no longer an advantage to survival, a much smaller percentage of blacks are affected.

More support for this fascinating theory comes from the significant fact that not only blacks, but other racial groups from the Middle Eastern and Mediterranean countries also sometimes possess the sickle-cell trait, though it occurs with less frequency than in blacks. (These groups include Italians, Greeks, and those of Near Eastern and Indian descent.) Among the blacks of South Africa, where there is little malaria, sickle-cell anemia is relatively rare.

There is little doubt that the slave trade of the sixteenth to eighteenth centuries helped spread the sickle-cell gene from Africa to the rest of the world. In the United States today the sickle-cell trait can be found in about 10 percent of the black population. About 1 in every 625 newborn black babies has sickle-cell anemia, and the disease is thought to affect between 25,000 and 50,000 persons in the United States alone.

Up to this point we have already mentioned both sickle-cell anemia and the sickle-cell trait. What is the difference between the two, and how are they related?

Sickle-cell anemia is a serious, often lethal disease that can be both extremely painful and very expensive for its victims. It is only one of the many hereditary blood diseases that is caused by abnormal hemoglobin. Hemoglobin is the reddish, iron-containing blood pigment that is responsible for carrying the life-giving oxygen to each of the cells in our bodies. This hemoglobin is concentrated in the disc-shaped red blood cells that give blood its characteristic color. Through a microscope red blood cells can be seen as doughnut-shaped discs, with thin centers and thick edges.

But the red blood cells of the victims of sickle-cell disease are grossly distorted and occur in pointed, elongated shapes which are reminiscent of crescents or sickles. This is how Dr. James Herrick, of Chicago, named the disease as he did. In 1910, Dr. Herrick spotted the sickled cells in the blood of a twenty-year-old West Indian student who had been complaining of cough, chills, fever, and dizziness.

In 1949 Nobel laureate Dr. Linus Pauling and his colleagues showed that the basis of the sickle-cell problem was a defect in the hemoglobin molecule itself.

The sickled cells are themselves characteristic of the problems this disease causes. Their pointy, sickled shape makes it difficult for them to move through the body's tiny blood vessels as easily as the normal red blood cells, which are bouncy and flexible. The sickled cells bump and snag, and pile up in clumps, which clog the capillaries and cause oxygen starvation in the tissues throughout the body. This often results in episodes of severe pain, called sickle-cell crises. During a crisis the pain may occur in the back, the abdomen, or in another specific part of the body. Sickle-cell crises are usually of limited duration, but they often require hospitalization and emergency treatment in the form of frequent blood transfusions. Sickle-cell crises can kill their victims.

To complicate matters, the body's natural mechanisms act quickly to remove the abnormal sickled cells from the bloodstream. Generally these imperfect red blood cells are removed faster than they can be replaced, and severe anemia is a result.

Thus, the victims of sickle-cell disease show the usual symptoms of severe anemia, including poor general development, with a short body trunk and long arms and legs. "Many patients," according to descriptions distributed by the National Institutes of Health,

> are moderately jaundiced, the whites of their eyes turning greenish-yellow. Chronic "punched out"-looking ulcers often appear about the ankles, along with a pallor in the palms of the hands, lips, nailbeds, and tissue linings of the mouth. Severe pain in the abdomen, and in the knees, elbows and other joints is experienced from time to time in almost all patients with the disease.
>
> In more severe cases, other symptoms include weakness, headache, dizziness, ringing in the ears and spots before the eyes. Patients are sometimes drowsy and irritable. Some patients have become used to their chronic anemia and in spite of some weakness can carry on daily activities except during painful episodes.

With all these varied symptoms, sickle-cell anemia can be confused with a wide variety of diseases. When one medical team reviewed 214 cases of sickle-cell anemia, they found that an incorrect diagnosis was made in 97 cases, or almost 50 percent. The disease was mistaken for appendicitis, peritonitis due to perforated ulcer, rheumatic fever, osteomyelitis, syphilis, pneumonia, encephalitis, and arthritis, among others.

For a long while it was thought that few victims of sickle-cell anemia survived to the third or fourth decades of life. But a 1966 report from the World Health Organization concluded:

> There is considerable variability in the life span of patients with [sickle-cell anemia] in various parts of the world. Early mortality appears to be the rule in East and

Central Africa, but longer survivals are observed in West Africa and the West Indies. In the U.S.A. survival into adult life is common.

Nevertheless, sickle-cell anemia kills many of its victims while they are very young. The disease, in fact, is almost always more severe in childhood, and those victims who survive to later life generally find the problem of the disease less severe. Many adults who have sickle-cell anemia carry on full-time jobs in spite of the disease.

The person who is found to have the sickle-cell *trait*, sometimes referred to as sicklemia, is *not* a victim of sickle-cell anemia, but is a carrier of a gene for this disease. As a matter of fact, the carriers of the sickle-cell trait usually don't even know about it (the same is true with regard to carriers of other recessive diseases). Dr. Howard Pearson stresses that "the person with sickle-cell trait should consider himself normal."

Today, effective blood tests for screening the sickle-cell trait exist. At the present time, however, no reliable prenatal tests have yet been perfected to determine whether the fetus is a victim of sickle-cell disease. There is a strong possibility that such a test will be developed in the future.

As in the case of Tay Sachs disease, therefore, carriers of the sickle-cell trait can be spotted by medical scientists. But unlike Tay Sachs disease, sickle-cell anemia can't be detected *in utero*. Thus, there is no viable follow-up to the screening other than the choices of either not marrying another carrier of the trait, avoiding having children altogether, or proceeding with your family and taking the calculated risk that they will not inherit the disease.

If you are a black person, you may be at risk for sickle-cell anemia. A simple blood test can determine whether you are a carrier.

If both you and your spouse are found to be carriers of the sickle-cell trait, each of your children has a one-in-four chance of having sickle-cell anemia; one chance in two of only carrying the trait (as you do); and one chance in four of being absolutely free of the sickle-cell trait.

If only one parent has the sickle-cell trait, none of the children will have sickle-cell anemia, but each child has a 50-percent chance of carrying the trait.

If one parent has sickle-cell anemia and the other parent is free of both the disease and the trait, all children will carry the trait, but none can actually inherit sickle-cell anemia.

If one parent has sickle-cell anemia, and the other parent has the sickle-cell trait, all of their children will have either sickle-cell anemia or the sickle-cell trait.

It is hopeful that a safe and effective prenatal test for sickle-cell anemia will be available within the next few years.

HEMOPHILIA

Hemophilia, also known as the "bleeder's disease," or the "disease of royalty," was possibly the first inherited disease known to man *as* an inherited disease. We have already mentioned how hemophilia is even referred to in the ancient Babylonian Talmud.

As with so many rare and serious diseases there are a lot of old wives' tales and other misconceptions about hemophilia. Most people think, for example, that since the hemophiliac is "a bleeder," that the smallest cut, scratch, or even a pinprick will lead to severe and probably fatal episodes of bleeding.

In fact, this is not the case. Dr. C. Casper has explained,

> When a hemophiliac is injured, he does not bleed harder or faster than normal, but he keeps on bleeding because he can't make a firm clot to plug the torn blood vessels. Small cuts on the skin are usually not a problem, but bleeding in any deeper area is prolonged. Some bleeding episodes occur as a result of obvious trauma, but many occur seemingly without cause. Normal persons may often rupture small vessels in various tissues due to slight strains, but a clot forms quickly and the person is never aware of the episode.

Thus the real danger to the victim of hemophilia is not the small cut on a finger, but the deeper—and therefore more difficult to quickly spot—blood vessel damage that may continue for days. This kind of bleeding can result in severe bruises, and extensive bleeding into muscles and joints can occur. If such bleeding into the joints happens frequently, a kind of deforming arthritis can develop, as well as weakness in muscles adjacent to the affected joints. Severe pain often accompanies the episodes of internal bleeding.

Hemophilia is a sex-linked disease. You will recall that we explained the mechanisms of sex linkage back in Chapter 2. Because of this type of inheritance, hemophilia can be "hidden" in carrier females for several generations, and then suddenly an affected male child will be born. (There have been only about sixty cases of known female hemophiliacs in all of recorded history. Usually, in order for a woman hemophiliac to be born, a male victim would have to impregnate a female carrier of the disease. Even then there is only a 50-percent chance of a daughter being a hemophiliac.)

It is also possible for a woman to bear a hemophilic child with absolutely no family history of the disease, since a third or more of all hemophilia patients represent a new genetic mutation.

When a carrier mother and a normal father have children, there is a 50-percent risk that any male offspring will have hemophilia (50-percent chance for males to have hemophilia; 50-percent chance for a normal male; 50-percent chance for a normal girl; 50-percent chance for a carrier girl).

As we have stressed before, these odds remain the same with each pregnancy, and the birth of one affected son does not in any way ameliorate the chances of subsequent children being affected by the disease. Families exist which have only one hemophilic boy and one or more normal youngsters, yet other families have two, three, or even four hemophilic sons.

Hemophilia became known as "the royal disease," because Queen Victoria of England (1819–1901) was a carrier. One of her sons had hemophilia; two of her daughters—and several granddaughters—also carried the disease. As Victoria's affected descendants married into the royal families throughout Europe, the hidden hemophilia gene began to make itself known. One of Victoria's granddaughters was Alexandra, who married Czar Nicholas II of Russia and bore their son Alexis in 1904. Alexis was a victim of hemophilia. The story of Nicholas and Alexandra and their hemophilic son is a classic today, mainly because of the best-selling book by Robert Massie. Massie's interest in the royal Russian family came about partially because his own son is a victim of hemophilia. The family's story is told in the book *Journey,* written by Massie and his wife Suzanne.

In the case of the Russian Romanovs, the royal parents' anguished reactions to their son's profound illness led them to an unusual relationship with the monk Rasputin. This relationship no doubt affected the course of Russian history significantly, and, therefore, doubtlessly altered the modern history of the entire world.

In spite of such royal connections, however, hemophilia is not really a "royal" disease at all. It can, and does, strike ordinary individuals—mainly men—without regard to race or ethnic background.

When a person is a victim of hemophilia, his blood plasma lacks one of the proteins necessary to form a clot. Some researchers today believe that the necessary proteins are not actually missing, but they are inactive in their usual role. In the classic variety of hemophilia, also called hemophilia A, the missing protein is called AHF or factor VIII. Another form of the disease is called Christmas disease, or hemophilia B, and the missing protein in this disease is called PTC or factor IX.

There are as yet no known cures for hemophilia, but effective treatments have been developed. Such treatments are based upon concentrates of the missing "clotting factor," which can be isolated from the blood plasma of healthy donors. Infusions of this factor can be given to hemophiliacs either regularly as a preventive measure against hemorrhaging, or as needed whenever a "bleed" is occurring or may occur. The clotting factor can be self-administered, and can be carried along on trips, hence allowing a young man to go away to college and to become fairly independent. This is a giant stride from the days when there was virtually no hope for victims of hemophilia.

Treatment with the clotting factor, however, is so expensive that hemophilia has actually become the most expensive chronic disease in the United States, with costs for the clotting factor alone ranging between $6,000 and $26,000 per year.

Unfortunately, there are no completely accurate medical tests at this time which can detect carriers of hemophilia. Neither are there any prenatal diagnostic tests to determine whether a fetus is a victim of hemophilia.

However, if a family knows itself to be at risk for hemophilia there is one available alternative. Amniocentesis can be performed during pregnancy to determine whether the fetus is male or female. If the fetus is female, the pregnancy can be continued without worry of the child being a victim of hemophilia. If, however, the fetus is shown to be a male, the parents may decide upon termination of the pregnancy instead of taking a chance on having a child who suffers hemophilia. The risk inherent in making this choice, of course, is that there is a possibility that a normal male fetus will be aborted.

If the fetus is known to be female, and the disease itself, therefore, is not a worry, parents should be well aware of the possibility that their daughter might be a carrier of the disease. If this is the case, the parents will want to be sure to inform their daughter about this possibility so that she, too, will be able to make use of all the available medical knowledge and techniques when the time comes for her to become a mother herself.

If a woman who is at risk for bearing a hemophilic child is near the time of giving birth and has not had the opportunity to take advantage of special counseling and the tests we just discussed, she should be sure to inform her physician that there is a possibility the child will have hemophilia. Then, if the child is a boy, the doctors will be able to take a blood sample from the umbilical cord at birth to test for the disease. If the test is not performed at this time, there may be a wait of several months, until enough blood can be taken to test the child to see if he is afflicted.

A couple is known to be at risk for bearing a child with hemophilia if:

1 / The husband (or wife) is a hemophiliac.
2 / There is any history of hemophilia in the background of the wife's side of the family—father, grandfathers, uncles or cousins.

There is no significant risk of bearing a child with hemophilia if the father *is healthy,* but some of his relatives are victims of hemophilia.

CHAPTER

9

A
MATTER
OF
ETHICS

THE STRIKING ADVANCES IN HUMAN GENETICS DURING RE-
cent years have brought with them new ethical and
moral problems never before encountered either by
health professionals or their patients.

New technologies in all health care fields have provided us with increasing control over our lives, deaths,
and births. Some self-styled moralists today would carefully warn each of us that we "must not play God . . .
that only He has the right and the ability to make such
decisions . . ."

How quickly they have forgotten. We have been
"playing God" with regard to our lives and our health
for years.

Our medicines and machines have kept alive those
who, if Nature had her way, would have died long ago.
There are, to name a few, the diabetics, to whom we

provide insulin; the hemophiliacs, to whom we provide the clotting factor; the millions of victims of once-fatal infections, to whom we provide lifesaving antibiotics.

So, these life-and-death decisions are nothing new to us. As the technologies improve, however, we are faced with increasingly difficult choices, and we must make them far more often.

In no field do such decisions arise as frequently as they do in human genetics. In this final chapter we intend to raise some of the major ethical issues involved in genetic care today. There will be some answers, but many more questions. These are the questions with which all of us may someday have to cope. In spite of what some people say, the answers to these questions must not be left solely to the health care professionals, the clergymen, or the legislators, since it is *our* lives, and the lives of our families, that are directly affected.

ECONOMICS OF GENETICS

In some unfortunate families as many as 50 percent of the members may suffer profound genetic diseases. Health economists have estimated that fully 20 percent of the total cost of health care in the United States is accounted for by genetic disease.

Dr. J. E. Seegmiller of the University of California explains how this occurs:

The fact that many victims of hereditary disease are completely unable to care for themselves and require full-time care by their relatives or become lifetime wards of the state in mental institutions or nursing homes makes the total cost to the nation far greater than that of the diseases that kill (more or less) outright, such as cancer, stroke, or heart disease which usually affect individuals who have already lived out the major portions of their lives as contributing members of society.

It is obvious, therefore, that prenatal diagnosis of genetic disease, and genetic counseling, are legitimate and widespread medical needs. There is little doubt that, as in the case of other similar needs, the federal government will end up paying a good part of the bill for research, development, and actual practice.

Opponents of such federal or state programs have argued that massive genetic counseling and genetic screening programs may not be worthwhile. The facts show, however, that even when one boils it right down to the hard, cold dollars involved, well-planned and carefully executed genetic public health programs are well worth their expense.

It has been calculated, for example, that it costs a quarter of a million dollars to provide a lifetime of institutionalized care to a profoundly defective individual—that's a lifetime of *maintenance-level* care. Couple this with the fact that there are between 3,000 and 5,000 new babies with Down syndrome born in the United States every year. Quick calculations show that the annual money committed for merely maintaining these human beings in institutions is about $1 billion— and this figure represents only a single disease.

A child born with Tay Sachs disease, which affects mainly Jewish people descended from Eastern European stock, will live five years at most. Yet intensive care for each child born with this disease will cost as much as $50,000 per year. If, for example, 50 children were born with this rare disease in the United States every year, the annual cost for caring for the children with Tay Sachs disease born in a single year alone would come to at least two and a half million dollars.

Far more common is phenylketonuria, called PKU. This is a genetic disease that causes mental retardation because of a complex error in the child's metabolism. PKU occurs about once in every 14,000 births. It costs about $1.25 to screen each newborn baby for PKU; thus, it costs a great deal of money—$17,000—to detect each PKU victim at birth. Then another $8,000 to $16,000 must be spent for special dietary treatment for this child during the next five to ten years to prevent the disease from causing severe retardation. Thus the total cost for preventing PKU is about $33,000 for each affected child. It sounds expensive. But if untreated, the PKU victim would be profoundly retarded and would then spend perhaps fifty years in an institution. Cost: about $20 per day or roughly $365,000 for a lifetime— more than ten times the cost of prevention!

Many states and cities already have developed laws which require screening for one or more hereditary conditions at birth. The infant's participation in the tests is simple—just a needle-prick on the baby's heel and a few drops of blood collected on a special kind of paper. The bloodstained paper is sent to a laboratory where tests for more than half-a-dozen severe hereditary conditions can be carried out.

All of these examples, of course, are merely the "bare

bones" economics of a few genetic diseases. The actual impact of a successful genetic screening and counseling program is much greater, considering that each child who is successfully treated for a genetic disease can become a productive member of society, taking a job, earning a wage, paying taxes, and perhaps even making important social or intellectual contributions to the world in which he lives.

ABORTION

The complicated ethical and moral question of abortion is highly relevant to genetic counseling and genetic disease, for obvious reasons. Since no cures have yet been discovered for the vast majority of genetic diseases, the most practical way to combat them is for people to avoid having children with major genetic defects.

In those circumstances in which it is possible to detect these defects in a fetus, the only way to avoid actually bearing the child with the disease is abortion. The vast majority of individuals consider the destruction of a diseased fetus far more acceptable than the destruction of an individual who already has been born, no matter what the age.

A great deal has been written about the moral implications of deciding when human life actually begins. Some people believe life occurs at the moment that the egg and sperm unite, and that any interference with the growth process is to be considered the destruction of a viable human life.

Others, however, insist that human life begins when

the fetus "quickens," or begins to move, about twenty weeks after conception. Yet another group believes that human life starts only upon the separation of the fetus from the mother and the beginning of its independent existence.

There are compelling arguments on all sides of the controversy of exactly when human life actually begins, and each of these arguments has its validity. There seems to have been, however, much less discussion and consideration of the human consequences that result when the decision is made—usually on moral or ethical grounds—not to allow abortion of a genetically diseased fetus.

Although, in human terms, the consequences of such decisions are actually immeasurable, we do know that regardless of the ethical, moral, or religious bases of the decision, the effect on individual families is usually staggering. Elsewhere in this book we have discussed some of the biological and psychological implications of people's reproductive lives. Now we must turn to some of the less clearly defined ethical and moral ramifications of these problems.

Even irreligious families, when faced with an extreme personal crisis such as a complicated pregnancy, will often turn to their church for guidance and comfort. Many religious groups have considered and accepted the necessity of some form of birth control, but they have been less definitive in their regulations concerning abortion, especially when a profoundly defective fetus is the reason for the abortion.

This attitude on the part of some religious groups can

be exemplified by Mrs. Smith, a Catholic, who unexpectedly became pregnant at age forty-two. Because of
her age she was referred by her obstetrician to a medical center in a large western state for a complete genetic
evaluation and amniocentesis.

Mrs. Smith was also concerned about this surprise
pregnancy, and she shared her physician's opinion that
her situation needed a careful medical evaluation. Early
in the counseling process, it was explained to Mrs. Smith
that if she happened to be carrying a severely defective
child she would probably have only one option if she
wanted to do something about it. That option would
be to have an abortion.

The fact is, however, that most women firmly believe
that tests will show that they are not carrying a defective
baby (indeed, this is what most tests *do* reveal). Thus
women about to undergo prenatal procedures are not
usually reluctant to say they will consider having an
abortion if a problem is discovered. For this reason,
many physicians who perform prenatal diagnoses no
longer insist that the mothers agree in advance to consider abortion if a defective fetus is found. These physicians have learned from experience that only the reality
of knowing that the child they are carrying suffers from
a profound disease or deformity will enable the parents
to make a truly informed decision.

Mrs. Smith was in exactly this position, and when
prenatal tests showed the presence of Down syndrome
in the fetus, she panicked, and neither she nor her husband was able to make a decision regarding abortion.

The members of the genetics team which had prepared her for the tests and carried them out were not surprised by this reaction. They spent long hours with the parents, discussing the various possibilities and options open to them. As professionals in the counseling field the genetics team was especially concerned with trying to present to the parents a fair and realistic picture of what they and their other children might expect if Mrs. Smith delivered this Down syndrome baby. At the same time, they wanted Mrs. Smith to fully understand what to expect from an abortion, if that was the decision she made.

In the course of her deliberations, Mrs. Smith turned to her priest for religious counseling. He told her quite simply that abortion was morally wrong and there were *no* circumstances which would warrant the destruction of her unborn baby's life. While the priest was kind in his delivery of this edict, he did not ask Mrs. Smith any questions about the life of her family, or their capacity to care for a child with such a severe problem.

Such advice from the clergy is considered by some to be an indication of great strength and moral stamina. But one might rightly ask, whose strength and stamina does it really demonstrate? How many religious authorities offering such advice are concerned with the physical, emotional, or financial burdens the result of their advice places on a family? How many fully appreciate the terribly damaged quality of the life they so strenuously recommend bringing to term?

In Mrs. Smith's case, and in others like it, the church appears to have added another kind of burden to the one this family was already trying to face. And, indeed,

Mrs. Smith made the difficult decision to carry her baby to term, for she was unable to accept the moral stigma which her church would have placed on her if she had the abortion. We believe that decisions of this magnitude should be made solely by the parents, who will be responsible for such a child.

Sumner Twiss, Jr., an instructor in Brown University's Department of Religious Studies, has noted that:

> . . . parents are in the best and perhaps a unique position to assess the total impact that a genetically defective child may have on themselves and their families. The fetal right to life, if there be such, does not override the parental right, for it may be plausibly argued that a fetus possesses a serious right to life only if it has the potentiality to become a self-conscious being, capable of self-determination and free agency. This condition is absent in the case of many genetic conditions.

It is true, after all, that rights and obligations are dependent upon each other, and unless one has the obligation to maintain a profoundly diseased child, one should probably not have the right—morally or ethically —to determine whether such a life should exist. The parents, of course, should have access to all kinds of unbiased advice in making their decisions—from physicians, social workers, psychologists, as well as from clergymen.

For Mrs. Smith, the decision to bring her Down syndrome baby to term was agonizing. It was clear to the medical staff caring for her that she was in deep conflict about her final decision to deliver this child.

She was especially distraught about the effect the new

child might have on her other four children, to whom she had an established, well-defined commitment. Both Mr. and Mrs. Smith were painfully concerned that their decision to give birth to a retarded child was not only a commitment for the rest of their lives, but that they were also possibly condemning their four children to sharing the lifelong responsibility for the new sibling, who would, indeed, be dependent for a lifetime.

The aunt of a young girl with Down syndrome observed:

> . . . loving though one may be, I assure you that the work is endless and monumentally taxing. Parents of mongoloids are not always comfortably off, and the sheer drudgery grinds them down. To knowingly bring such a baby into the world imposes on it a precarious existence and on others crushing responsibilities.

Adds Dr. F. Clarke Fraser, professor of medical genetics at McGill University, "I think it would have to be a very 'warm and loving' couple that would not suffer from the birth of a mongoloid child. Some families I know have made a noble adjustment to their tragedy, but not without suffering."

The conflict over selective abortion develops when parents like the Smiths understandably place a higher value on their desire for a normal child than on a defective one. This value judgment is logical and understandable to most parents. But it is not acceptable to religious groups which depend strictly upon the biblical commandments to procreate and do not really consider the quality of a particular life. Even in the case of the invariably fatal Tay Sachs disease, strict Orthodox Jewish law does not allow the element of choice in the matter of procreation.

In such situations the orthodox religious viewpoint does not allow for an important distinction. When abortion is considered because of genetic need, it is not simply a matter of convenience. Instead, this alternative is chosen to avoid bringing into the world a child with a severe genetic abnormality who is thus destined to an inevitably tragic life.

At this time, no devout religious group has been able to adjust its ethical and philosophical values to meet the needs of parents facing this tragic conflict. Parents will surely question themselves about the purpose of saving a child who is genetically destined—as is the case in Tay Sachs disease, for example—to die a certain death within only a few years of birth. But there will be no acceptable answer to them in their dual role as religious persons and as parents.

The depth of this conflict is so severe that even some physicians, who know very well the fate of these children, are recommending that they be "saved." One of them, Dr. Fred Rosner, has stated that "Human beings should not be reproduced or manufactured, but 'called into being' and given the breath of life by Divine intervention."

Dr. Rosner interprets this concept of life to mean that the destruction of a fetus is unacceptable for any reason whatsoever.

We believe this judgment can never be justified when weighed against the feelings of those who believe that, in certain circumstances, parents may have the duty to avoid bearing children with serious genetic defects, if possible.

AMNIOCENTESIS AND PRENATAL DIAGNOSIS

Another important area of ethical concern is prenatal diagnosis, particularly amniocentesis. As we have already mentioned, the procedure is recommended for all pregnant women older than thirty-five years, as well as for women who have borne children with other inborn errors of metabolism for which testing is possible.

Although the procedure carries a risk of only .5 percent, it does not appear warranted to assume even that minimal risk unless the mother has decided she will have an abortion if a defective fetus is found. What, after all, is the point of knowing that one is going to bear a profoundly diseased child, unless something is going to be done about it?

However, a growing number of specialists in human genetics are of the opinion that parents have the right to know every bit of available information about the child they are expecting, regardless of any decisions they might make about terminating the pregnancy. But a related problem involves the still limited availability of testing resources at the present time. Should a parent who has definitely decided against having an abortion, even if the fetus is defective, be given equal priority in access to testing facilities as the parent who has decided to have an abortion if the prenatal tests show a severe genetic disease? There is evidence that parents cannot make such decisions in the abstract and that the known presence of a defective fetus can result in parents reversing their previous objection to abortion.

Naturally, the opinions that parents have with regard to amniocentesis and subsequent abortion will often reflect the attitudes of their physicians. When, for example, a physician is not convinced that prenatal diagnosis is warranted for a particular patient, he may present the .5-percent risk inherent in amniocentesis as a high risk, thus discouraging the mother from undergoing the procedure. There have been documented reports of obstetricians whose religious beliefs do not encompass the possibility of abortion and who, therefore, have simply decided not to offer prenatal diagnosis to their patients. Today, these physicians are obligated, both ethically and professionally, to refer appropriate patients to other expert physicians who do not have the same moral conflicts.

THE COUNSELOR

Special consideration must be given to the role played by the genetic counselor in helping families determine their genetic risks and how to handle them. These counselors are usually consulted with the expectation that both a diagnosis and a medical plan will be recommended.

Likewise, many families are referred by their own physicians for consultation services with a geneticist, and often this includes the services of an entire team of counselors. The assumption in this case, of course, is that the team will develop a recommended plan of action for the parents.

But the counselors, too, are increasingly careful not to impose their own ideas and prejudices on their clients. This often results in confusion for the patient and even for the referring physician, both of whom expect definitive answers to the problems at hand.

All genetic counselors have been faced with the question, "What would you do in my situation?" Some counselors will honestly tell the patient what his or her decision would be. Other counselors will reply that since they are not personally facing the dilemma, they cannot honestly supply an appropriate answer. Such counselors usually make every effort to assure themselves that their patients understand all facets of the problem, and strive to present all sides as objectively as possible. These counselors understand that they can have a tremendous influence over their patients, who are particularly vulnerable since they often do not fully grasp the role inheritance plays in the formation of disease.

This puts the patients in the position of having to make the decisions for themselves, based on their understanding of the situation. While this approach is usually relatively successful, many counselors are concerned lest the patient nevertheless be influenced by the opinion of the person offering the counseling.

It is, of course, possible that sometimes a counselor may feel that a particular course of action is the "right" one for a particular client. The effect of such a reaction by the counselor is usually subtle, since professional counselors learn to diminish the influence of their own opinions on the actual counseling. Parents should, therefore, be alert to any undue influence their counselors may have on their perception of the genetic risks they face.

The counselor may well be prejudiced toward the very plan the parents themselves favor. Still, it is incumbent on the counselor to give the parents all the support needed to make such decisions on their own.

COMMUNICATING WITH FAMILY MEMBERS

Another potentially troublesome question deals with the obligation of a patient discovered to have an inherited condition to inform other members of his or her family that they may also be at risk for the disease.

When the disease is one that can be treated, the reasons for informing family members are more positive than when knowledge of the defect can bring only anxiety.

Most often there are compelling reasons to share the knowledge of any hereditary condition with other family members, since there always exists the possibility that treatment for the disease may become available in the future. When families are still in their reproductive years it would be genuinely irresponsible to withhold the information which could allow them to prevent the birth of a defective child.

Some individuals, however, have great difficulty in sharing information about inherited diseases with their relatives, because they suffer from the severe guilt and embarrassment which often accompanies the presence of such conditions. Guilt and shame are exacerbated, however, by failure to share the information. Experience has also shown that families are rarely able to keep such kinds of secrets to themselves, and that the energy exerted in denying these facts is much more wisely spent in actually confirming and dealing with their existence. Once a person or family accepts the biological truth that they are not personally responsible for any hereditary disease they or their family members may suffer, they may be able to help other family members reach a proper understanding of the situation.

When parents know their children may be carriers of a specific defective gene, they may be especially vulnerable to the impulse to keep this information from the children. Often, out of ignorance rather than malice, parents will then reveal such information at the worst possible time and when the son or daughter is least able to manage it. This frequently occurs when a young person announces that he or she plans to marry, for example.

Girls who have brothers with hemophilia are often not aware that they, too, may be carriers of this sex-linked defective gene. They, in turn, may transmit the disease to their own sons.

While knowledge of this possibility is not simple to live with—and no one can easily advise mothers exactly when and how to discuss such matters with their daughters—there is absolutely no doubt that children are entitled to this kind of information about themselves.

Withholding such knowledge can be far more destructive than sharing it with each child at the proper time.

A young woman with such a known risk can, by the time she has married, have come to accept herself as a potential parent even with her liability. She and her husband will have learned a lot about dealing with their fears and disappointments in advance of the event, if it occurs. They will already have had the opportunity—possibly with expert guidance—to understand their risk, both medically and in terms of their parental expectations. They will be able to choose a course of action based upon their own hopes and solid basic information.

Experience indicates that individuals who have been informed about potential genetic problems in themselves and their families usually can reach a calm and logical decision when they are given the facts. It is only in rare instances that people react quickly, irrationally, or hysterically, and feel threatened that they are "bad," "unworthy," or "diseased" people. In most cases the ultimate decision made by individuals who have been given the facts—whether to avoid male children by aborting male fetuses following positive prenatal diagnosis, or to proceed with pregnancy—stands a good chance of being the right decision for this particular family.

SEX SELECTION

In view of the fact that prenatal diagnosis such as amniocentesis can reveal the sex of the fetus, there has been some concern over the use of such techniques solely for sex determination, since parents sometimes prefer children of one sex rather than the other.

In the case of a sex-linked disease—hemophilia, for example—the detection of the sex of the fetus is crucial to the decision the parents may make. Since only males have such diseases (except in extremely rare instances), parents who could possibly pass this disease to their offspring may choose to abort all male fetuses. As there is no prenatal test at this time to detect most of the sex-linked diseases, there is always a 50-percent chance of aborting a healthy male fetus. In spite of this, the choice of abortion for possibly affected male fetuses is seen by most genetic health professionals as a legitimate one.

On the other hand, with the same prenatal diagnostic techniques it is possible for parents to ask for the abortion of an unaffected fetus simply because it is not of the desired sex.

It is true that genetic selection of any kind makes people uncomfortable because of the political implications inherent in any capability for choosing "good people," over those who are "less good," according to an arbitrary set of standards. For the most part, however, geneticists are committed to helping people select healthy babies over babies who are known to be unhealthy. To this end, amniocentesis is valuable, since the modest risks of amniocentesis for mother and child are much lower than the possible burden of bearing a severely ill child under most circumstances.

But a mother who has no major chance of bearing a genetically diseased child, and simply seeks to know the sex of the fetus she carries, is placing both herself and her child at unnecessary risk because of the medical procedures that need to be carried out. Such a parent, too, will possibly affect the natural distribution of males and females, which may not make much of a difference . on an individual basis, but if carried out across the world could have serious ramifications for the future of the human race.

Also of interest to this discussion is the fact that the parent who requests medical procedures to predetermine a child's sex will be using medical and technological expertise which is presently in short supply, thus perhaps depriving a family at risk for genetic disease of these vital services.

These various factors will continue to cause stress as an increasing number of parents, perhaps without understanding the profound implications of what they seek, become knowledgeable about the possibility of prenatal sex determination.

SCREENING FOR
GENETIC DISEASE

Voluntary screening of particular populations for genetic diseases has been practiced for several years. This kind of screening can be done on a large scale and the benefits can be significant. The potential dangers of such a program, however, are equally significant.

One of the first mass screening programs, for example, was aimed at discovering the sickle-cell trait, which affects about 10 percent of American blacks. Unfortunately lack of experience in such programs led to a poorly planned and executed screening of the many people involved, with the result that many blacks subsequently refused to participate in the programs. Prescreening education programs about sickle-cell disease were minimal, partly because of a shortage of trained health workers.

The result of all this was serious confusion in both the black and the white population.

Many blacks felt that sickle-cell disease and the sickle-cell trait were simply new ways to stigmatize black Americans. Blacks soon found, for example, that insurance firms were raising the premiums for carriers of the sickle-cell trait. Some employers were even restricting carriers of the sickle-cell trait from taking certain jobs on the grounds that their health was substandard. Even today sickle-cell carriers are barred from the Air Force Academy, but they are accepted at both Annapolis and West Point.

Since the incidence of both sickle-cell disease and the sickle-cell trait are high in the American black population, well-managed screening programs would seem to be an effective way to reduce the incidence of this disease. But unfortunately, the harmful effects of the previous, poorly organized and premature screening programs seem to have doomed such public health measures to failure. In spite of this unfortunate beginning, it is hoped that this particular failure will not prevent the black population from benefiting from the advantages such screening programs can offer, namely the information that enables couples to plan their families with full knowledge of any special risks they might face.

It is hoped that in the near future there will be a pre-natal test available which can diagnose a fetus with sickle-cell disease. Some black parents may want to abort an affected fetus in the hope that the next one will be unaffected. For such parents the knowledge that they are at risk for having a child with sickle-cell disease would be important to alert them to the need for amniocentesis. Today, however, when the prenatal test for sickle-cell disease is not yet available, some experts believe the reasons for screening may be cloudy.

Dr. Robert F. Murray, Jr., chief of the medical genetics program at Howard University College of Medicine, says: "In my view it doesn't really do patients a great deal of good to provide them with anxiety-provoking information that does not, at the same time, allow for some 'therapeutic' course of action."

Others argue that it is not necessarily a matter of therapeutic possibilities, but of the right to know one's reproductive potential. There are some parents who would rather not bear children at all, knowing they would in each case have a 25-percent chance of producing a child with a serious disease.

Professionals in the field of medical genetics have learned a good deal from the inadequacies of the sickle-cell screening program. Perhaps the major lesson has been that geneticists must be much more concerned about exactly how their scientific knowledge is trans-lated into public policy. Traditionally, physicians have not bothered much with such details. However, in the past, lack of understanding about sickle-cell disease and the sickle-cell trait certainly resulted in unnecessary stigmatization of carriers, many of whom suffered genuine economic and social consequences in the name of responsible health care.

Some experts have warned of dire consequences should any of the screening programs be made compulsory, especially in preschools or elementary schools. "It might happen that children identified as carriers could be stigmatized as different or as having undesirable parents or as being weaker or less fit," says Howard University's Dr. Robert Murray, Jr. "Furthermore, compulsory screening only in specific ethnic groups might also tend to reinforce racist doctrines."

Murray adds that "it is on the one hand unfair that everyone cannot yet know his or her 'mutant gene carrier status,' since all of us [are carriers of] at least several mutant genes, and also unfair that those whose mutant carrier status can be determined may be stigmatized by their peers."

While such problems may also attend future screening programs aimed at population groups at risk for rare diseases—such as Tay Sachs disease in Ashkenazic Jews and Cooley's anemia (thalassemia) for people of Mediterranean descent—it is important to realize that such dire consequences are certainly not inevitable. Increased knowledge of what can go wrong has also provided the opportunity to develop screening programs designed to avoid such failures.

Indeed, the major screening program for Tay Sachs disease, which started at about the same time as the screening for sickle-cell disease, was a huge success. The Tay Sachs program was first undertaken in Baltimore, and later in Washington, D.C., New York, and other cities, where great care was taken to educate those who were being screened. The screening tests were carried out only in areas where there were adequate facilities for follow-up on each case.

A major difference, of course, was the fact that at the time of these screening tests there already existed a reliable prenatal test for Tay Sachs disease. Thus, geneticists could virtually guarantee couples at risk for Tay Sachs disease that they could bear only normal children, so long as they agreed to abort any affected fetus.

Eventually, perhaps, similar testing situations will be developed for more common diseases, such as cystic fibrosis, which is the most prevalent genetic disease among American whites. With a test for CF available on a broad scale, many thousands of Americans could be told they are carrying a potentially deadly gene.

The ethical dilemma will be great, however, since cystic fibrosis no longer kills most of its young victims within a few years. Good medical care now allows cystic fibrosis patients to live well into their adult years. What will the parents-to-be of a child diagnosed in the womb as having cystic fibrosis want to do? Will abortion in such cases be justified?

Screening programs aimed at the so-called ethnic genetic diseases will no doubt continue to be politically controversial. However, even while the subject has been actively debated, there has been widespread screening of newborn infants for diseases such as phenylketonuria (PKU). These tests are quietly and automatically performed at birth in more than forty states in the nation. Their objective is specifically to reduce the incidence of this genetic disease, and the ensuing mental retardation.

In PKU the body is incapable of breaking down one of the common amino acids, called phenylalanine, which is found in many protein foods. Since the body cannot eliminate the amino acid, it accumulates and somehow causes severe mental retardation. When a newborn is found to have PKU, the child can promptly be placed on a diet very low in foods containing this particular amino acid. Such children are kept on this special diet until after their formative years of brain growth. The program has worked so well that, to date, many victims have been saved from tragic retardation. Ironically, however, additional problems have now arisen.

Women in whom PKU was discovered and successfully treated at birth are now having children of their own. It has been found that these children are often severely retarded, apparently affected by a toxic environment in the mother's uterus. This means that, in the case of females, newborns who are found to have PKU and are then put on the special diets must be followed for many years, so that when they become pregnant themselves they can again be put on the special diet.

What if these mothers-to-be do not want to go on the special diet? Considering the fact that society will probably have to bear the burden of caring for their profoundly retarded children, can such treatment be forced upon these women even if they don't want it?

Is it possible that someday people will have to undergo genetic screening tests before they are allowed to get married? Will certain marriages be barred? Will society be in a position to attempt to coerce certain individuals who are at risk for specific genetic diseases to forgo the right of having families of their own? Will forced sterilization for individuals who suffer from, or carry, certain genetic diseases become common? Who owns the information about our genetic shortcomings? Who should have access to it? Do our doctors have a duty to inform our relatives of what they find in our genes, since the relatives, too, may be affected? Or will the doctor who reveals such information be guilty of breaching the age-old rule of doctor-patient confidence? And what will happen when it becomes possible to detect in the womb not only the victims of certain genetic diseases, but also the carriers?

Will these frightening scenarios ever be acted out? Who can say? Some studies have already shown that even when individuals are found to be carriers of specific genetic diseases, the information doesn't significantly alter their choice of a marriage partner. Perhaps that is the way it should be. The big question then becomes whether such couples will plan their families with the genetic factor in mind.

In the long run, genetic medicine holds fantastic promise for reducing human suffering. It may not be easy to fulfill that promise because of the many pitfalls of this new and rapidly expanding branch of medicine.

The best chance for success lies in a broad program of public education about the factors involved in genetic counseling, so that when decisions are made—either on matters of private family concerns or on issues of public policy—the decisions will be based on complete information.

APPENDIX I

WHERE TO GET MORE INFORMATION ABOUT SPECIFIC GENETIC DISEASES

AMERICAN ACADEMY OF
PEDIATRICS
1801 Hinman Ave.
Evanston, IL 60204

AMERICAN COLLEGE OF
OBSTETRICIANS AND
GYNECOLOGISTS
79 West Monroe St.
Chicago, IL 60603

CENTER FOR SICKLE-CELL
ANEMIA
College of Medicine
Howard University
520 W Street NW
Washington, D.C. 20001

COMMITTEE TO COMBAT
HUNTINGTON'S DISEASE
200 West 57th St.
New York, NY 10019

COOLEY'S ANEMIA BLOOD AND
RESEARCH FOUNDATION
3366 Hillside Ave.
New Hyde Park, NY 11040

JOSEPH P. KENNEDY, JR.
FOUNDATION (MENTAL
RETARDATION)
Suite 205, 1701 K St. NW
Washington, D.C. 20006

MUSCULAR DYSTROPHY
ASSOCIATIONS OF AMERICA
1790 Broadway
New York, NY 10019

NATIONAL ASSOCIATION FOR
RETARDED CHILDREN
2709 Avenue E, East
Arlington, TX 76011

NATIONAL CYSTIC FIBROSIS
FOUNDATION
3379 Peachtree Road NE
Atlanta, GA 30326

NATIONAL FOUNDATION–
MARCH OF DIMES
P.O. Box 2000
White Plains, NY 10602

NATIONAL GENETICS
FOUNDATION
9 West 57th St.
New York, NY 10019

NATIONAL HEMOPHILIA
FOUNDATION
25 West 39th St.
New York, NY 10018

NATIONAL TAY SACHS AND
ALLIED DISEASES
ASSOCIATION, INC.
200 Park Avenue South
New York, NY 10003

UNITED STATES PUBLIC
HEALTH SERVICE
Public Information Officer
National Institutes of Health
Bethesda, MD 20014

APPENDIX II

STATE–BY–STATE LISTING OF GENETIC COUNSELING AND TREATMENT CENTERS

ALABAMA

Laboratory of Medical Genetics
University of Alabama Medical
  Center
Birmingham, Alabama 35294

Department of Medical
  Genetics
University of South Alabama
2451 Fillingim Street
Mobile, Alabama 36617

ALASKA

Dysmorphology Unit
1135 West 8th Ave.
Anchorage, Alaska

Public Health Service Genetics
  Clinics
University of Alaska
Box 95753
Fairbanks, Alaska 99701

ARIZONA

Genetic Counseling Center
St. Joseph's Hospital and
  Medical Center
P. O. Box 2071
Phoenix, Arizona 85001

College of Medicine, Obstetrics
  and Gynecology
The University of Arizona
Tucson, Arizona 85724

CALIFORNIA

Genetic Counseling Clinic
Kern County Health
  Department
Bakersfield, California 93305

Department of Medical
  Genetics
City of Hope National Medical
  Center
1500 East Duarte Road
Duarte, California 91010

Genetic Counseling Clinic
Valley Children's Hospital
Fresno, California 93703

Department of Pediatrics
University of California
  College of Medicine
Irvine, California 92650

Medical Genetics Unit
University of California,
  School of Medicine
La Jolla, California 92093

Department of Pediatrics,
  Genetics, Birth Defects &
  Chromosome Service
Loma Linda University
  Medical Center
Loma Linda, California 92354

Genetics Birth Defects Center
Los Angeles County–USC
  Medical Center
1129 North State St.
Los Angeles, California 90003

Division of Medical Genetics
Children's Hospital of
  Los Angeles
4650 Sunset Blvd.
Los Angeles, California 90054

Medical Genetics
Children's Hospital
Oakland, California 94609

Department of Pediatrics and
  Genetics
Kaiser Foundation Hospital
280 West MacArthur
  Boulevard
Oakland, California 94611

Department of Pediatrics
University of California, San
  Francisco Medical Center
San Francisco, California 94143

Genetic Counseling Clinic
San Luis Obispo County
  Health Department
2191 Johnson Ave.
San Luis Obispo, California
  93401

Genetic Counseling Clinic
Stanford University School of
  Medicine
Stanford, California 94305

Division of Medical Genetics
Harbor General Hospital
1000 West Carson St.
Torrance, California 90502

COLORADO

Genetics Unit
University of Colorado Medical
  Center
4200 East 9th Ave.
Denver, Colorado 80220

CONNECTICUT

Department of Pediatrics
University of Connecticut
  Health Center
Farmington, Connecticut 06032

Department of Human
  Genetics
Yale University School of
  Medicine
New Haven, Connecticut 06520

DELAWARE

Department of Pediatrics
Wilmington Medical Center
P. O. Box 1668
Wilmington, Delaware 20007

COUNSELING AND TREATMENT CENTERS

DISTRICT OF COLUMBIA

University Affiliated Center for
  Child Development
Georgetown University
  Medical Center
3900 Reservoir Road, NW
Washington, D.C. 20306

Division of Medical Genetics,
Department of Pediatrics
Howard University College of
  Medicine
Washington, D.C. 20001

Genetics Unit
Children's Hospital
Washington, D.C. 20009

FLORIDA

Birth Defects Center
University of Florida College
  of Medicine
Gainesville, Florida 32610

Mailman Center for Child
  Development
University of Miami School of
  Medicine
Miami, Florida 33152

GEORGIA

Department of Medical
  Genetics
Emory University School of
  Medicine
Atlanta, Georgia 30322

Birth Defects Center
Medical College of Georgia
Augusta, Georgia 30902

HAWAII

Department of Birth Defects
Kauikeolani Children's
  Hospital
Honolulu, Hawaii 96817

IDAHO

Idaho Department of Health
  and Welfare
State House
Boise, Idaho 83702

ILLINOIS

Amniocentesis Service
Michael Reese Hospital and
  Medical Center
530 East 31st St.
Chicago, Illinois 60616

Department of Pediatrics,
  Genetics, and Human
  Development
Rush Medical School
Rush-Presbyterian St. Luke's
  Medical Center
Chicago, Illinois 60612

Department of Genetics
Children's Memorial Hospital
Chicago, Illinois 60614

Genetics Counseling Service
University of Illinois
Urbana, Illinois 61801

Southern Illinois University
    School of Medicine
Springfield, Illinois 62708

INDIANA

Division of Medical Genetics
Indiana University Medical
    School
Indianapolis, Indiana 46207

IOWA

Department of Pediatrics
University Hospital
Iowa City, Iowa 52240

KANSAS

Division of Medical Genetics
Kansas University Medical
    School
Kansas City, Kansas 66103

KENTUCKY

Child Evaluation Center
University of Louisville
    Medical School
Louisville, Kentucky 40202

LOUISIANA

Department of Medicine,
    Section of Genetics
Louisiana State University
    School of Medicine
1542 Tulane Ave.
New Orleans, Louisiana 70112

Birth Defects Center
Louisiana State University
    School of Medicine
Shreveport, Louisiana 71130

MAINE

Maine Genetics Counseling
    Center
50 Union St.
Ellsworth, Maine 04605

Department of Pediatrics
Eastern Maine Medical Center
489 State St.
Bangor, Maine 04401

Birth Defects Clinic
Maine Medical Center
22 Branhall St.
Portland, Maine 04101

MARYLAND

The Moore Clinic
The Johns Hopkins Hospital
601 North Broadway
Baltimore, Maryland 21205

MASSACHUSETTS

Center for Genetic Counseling
and Birth Defects Evaluation
Tufts-New England Medical
Center
171 Harrison Ave.
Boston, Massachusetts 02111

Department of Pediatrics,
Genetics Unit
Massachusetts General
Hospital
Boston, Massachusetts 02114

Clinical Genetics Division
Children's Hospital Medical
Center
Boston, Massachusetts 02115

MICHIGAN

Department of Human
Genetics
University of Michigan
Medical Center
Ann Arbor, Michigan 48108

Birth Defects Center
Wayne State University
School of Medicine
275 East Hancock
Detroit, Michigan 48201

MINNESOTA

Human Genetics Clinic
University of Minnesota
Hospital
Minneapolis, Minnesota 55455

Department of Medical
Genetics
Mayo Clinic
Rochester, Minnesota 55901

MISSISSIPPI

Department of Preventive
Medicine
University of Mississippi
Medical Center
2500 North State St.
Jackson, Mississippi 39216

MISSOURI

Department of Pediatrics
Cardinal Glennon Memorial
Hospital
1465 South Grand Blvd.
St. Louis, Missouri 63104

Division of Medical Genetics
Washington University
Medical School
St. Louis, Missouri 63110

Genetic Counseling Center
Children's Mercy Hospital
Kansas City, Missouri 63104

MONTANA

Shodair Genetic and Birth
Defects Unit
840 Helena Ave.
Helena, Montana 59601

NEBRASKA

Center for Genetic Evaluation
Children's Memorial Hospital
Omaha, Nebraska 68105

NEW HAMPSHIRE

Department of Maternal and
Child Health
Dartmouth-Hitchcock Medical
Center
Hanover, New Hampshire
03755

NEW JERSEY

Department of Pediatrics
Hackensack Hospital
Hackensack, New Jersey 07601

Department of Pediatrics
New Jersey Medical School
100 Bergen St.
Newark, New Jersey 07103

NEW YORK

Birth Defects Institute
Albany Medical College
Albany, New York 12208

Genetic Counseling Program
Albert Einstein College of
Medicine
Bronx, New York 10461

Department of Pediatrics,
Medical Genetics Section
The Brookdale Hospital
Medical Center
Brooklyn, New York 11212

Division of Human Genetics
Children's Hospital of Buffalo
Buffalo, New York 14222

Division of Genetics
North Shore University
Hospital
Manhasset, New York 11030

Division of Genetics
College of Physicians and
Surgeons
Columbia University
New York, New York 10032

Division of Medical Genetics
Mount Sinai School of
Medicine
New York, New York 10029

Genetic Counseling Clinic
New York Hospital–Cornell
University Medical Center
New York, New York 10021

Division of Human Genetics
Long Island Jewish–Hillside
Medical Center
New Hyde Park, New York
11040

Division of Genetics
University of Rochester
  Medical Center
Rochester, New York 14642

Department of Pediatrics,
  Birth Defects Center
Westchester County Medical
  Center
Valhalla, New York 10595

NORTH CAROLINA

Genetic Counseling Service
University of North Carolina
  School of Medicine
Chapel Hill, North Carolina
  27514

Medical Genetics Section
Bowman Gray School of
  Medicine
Winston-Salem, North
  Carolina 27103

OHIO

Department of Pediatrics
Cleveland Metropolitan
  General Hospital
Cleveland, Ohio 44109

Genetics Center
Case Western Reserve
  University School of
  Medicine
Cleveland, Ohio 44106

Medical Genetics Section
Kettering Medical Center
Kettering, Ohio 45429

OKLAHOMA

Department of Pediatrics
University of Oklahoma
  Children's Hospital
Oklahoma City, Oklahoma
  73190

OREGON

Genetics Clinic
University of Oregon Medical
  School
Portland, Oregon 97201

PENNSYLVANIA

Division of Genetics
Jefferson Medical College
Philadelphia, Pennsylvania
  19107

Department of Human
  Genetics
University of Pennsylvania
  School of Medicine
Philadelphia, Pennsylvania
  19174

Department of Obstetrics,
  Gynecology, and Pediatrics
Magee-Women's Hospital
Pittsburgh, Pennsylvania
  15213

SOUTH CAROLINA

Section of Clinical Genetics,
  Department of Oral
  Medicine
Medical University of South
  Carolina
80 Barre St.
Charleston, South Carolina
  28401

Greenwood Genetic Center
1020 Spring St.
Greenwood, South Carolina
  29646

SOUTH DAKOTA

Medical Genetics Program
University of South Dakota
  Medical School
Vermillion, South Dakota
  57069

TENNESSEE

Birth Defects Evaluation
  Center
University of Tennessee
  Hospital
Knoxville, Tennessee 37916

Department of Pediatrics
University of Tennessee Center
  for Health Sciences
Memphis, Tennessee 38163

Medical Genetics Section,
  Department of Pediatrics
Meharry Medical College
Nashville, Tennessee 37208

TEXAS

Division of Medical Genetics
University of Texas,
  Southwestern Medical School
5323 Harry Hines Blvd.
Dallas, Texas 75235

Department of Pediatrics and
  Human Genetics
University of Texas Medical
  Branch
Galveston, Texas 77550

Section of Medical Genetics
Baylor College of Medicine
Houston, Texas 77025

Section of Genetics
University of Texas Medical
  School
7703 Floyd Curl Drive
San Antonio, Texas 78229

UTAH

Department of Internal
  Medicine
University of Utah College of
  Medicine
50 North Medical Drive
Salt Lake City, Utah 84112

COUNSELING AND TREATMENT CENTERS

VIRGINIA

Genetics Unit
University of Virginia School
of Medicine
Charlottesville, Virginia 22901

Department of Human
Genetics
Medical College of Virginia
Richmond, Virginia 23298

WASHINGTON

Department of Medicine
University of Washington
Seattle, Washington 98195

WEST VIRGINIA

Department of Medical
Genetics
West Virginia University
Medical Center
Morgantown, West Virginia
26506

WISCONSIN

Department of Medical
Genetics
University of Wisconsin
Medical School
Madison, Wisconsin 53706

PUERTO RICO

Sección de Genética Médica
Hospital Universitaria de
Niños
San Juan, Puerto Rico 00936

SELECTED
BIBLIOGRAPHY

Anthony, E. J. and Benedek, T. *Parenthood.* Boston: Little, Brown, 1970.

Bergsma, D., ed. Ethical, social and legal dimensions of screening for human genetic disease. *Original Article Series,* Vol. X, No. 6, 1974.

Deutsch, H. *The Psychology of Women.* 2 vols. New York: Grune and Stratton, 1945.

Ditzion, J., et al. *Our Bodies, Ourselves.* 2nd ed. New York: Simon and Schuster, 1976.

Duff, Raymond and Campbell, A. G. M. Moral and ethical dilemmas in the special-care nursery. *New Eng. J. Med.* *289*:890–4, 1973.

Erbe, Richard W. Current concepts in genetics: principles of medical genetics. *New Eng. J. Med. 294*:381, 480–2, 1976.

Fletcher, J. Attitudes toward defective newborns. *The Hastings Center Report 2,* January 1974.

Hilton, B., Callahan, D., Harris, M. and Condleffe, P., eds. *Ethical Issues in Human Genetics.* 1973.

Lynch, Henry T. *Dynamic Genetic Counseling for Physicians.* Springfield, Ill.: Charles C. Thomas, 1969.

Lynch, Patrick M. and Lynch, Henry T. Medical-legal aspects of familial cancer. *J. Leg. Med. 4(5)*:10–6, 1976.

McKusick, V. A. *Mendelian Inheritance in Man.* 4th ed. Baltimore: The Johns Hopkins Press, 1975.

Milunsky, A. *The Prevention of Genetic Disease and Mental Retardation.* Philadelphia: W. B. Saunders Company, 1975.

————. *Know Your Genes.* Boston: Houghton Mifflin Company, 1977.

National Research Council–National Academy of Sciences. *Genetic Screening: Programs, Principles, and Research.* Washington, D.C.: National Academy of Sciences, 1975.

Nyhan, William. *The Heredity Factor.* New York: Grosset and Dunlap, 1976.

Rosenstock, I. M., Childs, B. and Simopoulos, A. P. *Genetic Screening. A Study of the Knowledge and Attitudes of Physicians.* Washington, D.C.: National Academy of Sciences, 1975.

Shepard, T. H. *Catalogue of Teratogenic Agents.* 2nd ed. Baltimore: The Johns Hopkins Press, 1976.

Silman, Roberta. "The Bad Baby." In: *Blood Relations.* Boston: Little Brown, Atlantic, 1977.

Sutton, H. E. *An Introduction to Human Genetics.* 2nd ed. New York: Holt, Rinehart and Winston, 1975.

Todres, I. D., Krane, D., Howell, M., and Shannon, D. "Pediatricians' attitudes affecting decision-making in defective newborns." (In press.)

U.S. Department of Health, Education and Welfare. *What Are the Facts About Genetic Disease?* DHEW publication No. (NIH) 74-370. Bethesda, 1974.

Wexler, Nancy S. The counselor and genetic disease: Huntington's disease as a model. Paper presented at the meeting of the APA, Chicago, Ill., August 1975.

INDEX

INDEX

INDEX